"You were born FAT"

By Elizabeth Petruccione

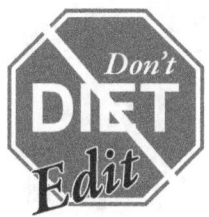

INTRODUCING
the 'Banking Method'
A practical and permanent way to lose weight

Elizabeth Petruccione battled her fat demons for more than forty years until she found herself under the layers and began her weight loss journey. After a 93 pound weight loss and three years of providing professional weight loss coaching with a national chain, Elizabeth opened the doors to weight loss for others with the founding of Losing Weight With Elizabeth...

203.756.2955
Blog: LosingWeightWithElizabeth.blogspot.com
Facebook: Losing Weight with Elizabeth
Email: losingweightwithelizabeth@gmail.com
Website: http://losingweightwithelizabeth

CONTENTS

INTRODUCTION

Probably as you are well aware, obesity in this country is reaching epidemic levels and costing our society billions of dollars in health related problems. So why are we one of the most obese nations? Much of it comes down to our lifestyle here in the United States. Most people do not realize that there are many "factors" involved with weight gain and weight loss for that matter. Oftentimes it's not just what we eat that is contributing to our obesity but factors such as stress, lack of activity and psychological factors that have been embedded in our subconscious minds.

Over the years there have been numerous "diets" that have come and gone. Probably too many to even count. Some have been extreme and wacky while others have been so simple with just one ingredient such as with the Grapefruit Diet.

If you're like most people who have tried to lose weight, you probably have tried many of these diets yourself without lasting results. Why? One of the simplest facts is that many of the so-called diets are not sustainable for extended periods of time. Sure, people will lose a few pounds short-term but typically end up gaining that weight back that they lost plus sometimes even a few more pounds in addition.

In this book, Elizabeth does a great job explaining and guiding you with examples of what it takes to lose weight, keep the weight off and maintain a healthier lifestyle. One of her key components to this program is her calorie "banking system." This system is similar to our monetary banking system but with calories instead. This concept is simple yet very powerful!

While it is great to lose weight you also have to remember is just as important to remain healthy. By implementing Elizabeth's recommendations, you potentially could lower your blood pressure, lower your cholesterol, improve your sex life, feel better about yourself and your appearance, have more confidence and finally lose the extra weight that's been nagging you for years.

Elizabeth is one of the best testimonials when it comes to her weight-loss program. She herself has lost 93 pounds over the past few years but the best part is that she has kept the weight off! Elizabeth knows firsthand how being overweight can increase your health risks. There was a time when she was on numerous medications for various health conditions. When she began losing weight, she also decreased her medication intake. Elizabeth is one of the most enthusiastic, positive and up beat person you will come across. There is no better weight-loss coach around. So pat yourself on your back for picking up this book and get ready to change your life for good!

Dr. Mike Swierczynski, DC, MS

CHAPTER ONE

BEGINNINGS

"You were born fat,"exclaimed my mother at least once a week for years. "You were born fat!" Just what every little girl wants to hear. In hindsight I'm certain I used those words as an excuse along with other excuses like "she's big boned" or "she has a thyroid condition." Such rationality always seemed to make the hurt just a little less hurtful. My mother wasn't far off base. I checked into this world at eight and a half pounds. That was about three pounds heavier than the average child born in 1948, the year of my birth. So maybe Mom was right. I was born fat. She believed it and certainly tried to convince me of that notion until the day she died. Mom also theorized that up to age eleven my weight was attributed to baby fat, and once I became a "woman," the baby fat would disappear.

By the time I was a teenager and the baby fat had not disappeared, my mother began to place me on numerous diets, the likes of which might seem Draconian by today's standards. Not that any "diet" isn't Draconian. More on that thought anon. Let's remember that diets in the 1960's were not as readily available as they are today and certainly not as healthy by any means. One such unhealthy diet my Mom assigned me to was called the *AYDS DIET*. The *AYDS DIET* was an appetite suppressant candy available in chocolate, chocolate mint, butterscotch or caramel flavors. The active ingredient in the AYDS candy was benzocaine, a local anesthetic commonly used as a topical pain reliever. The benzocaine was presumably used to reduce the sense of taste to reduce eating. The product name was changed to Diet Ayds in the early 1980's but eventually vanished from the market place as people began to identify it with *Aids - acquired immune deficiency syndrome.*

I was also placed on a very early version of the *ATKINS*, low carb diet then known as *THE STILLMAN DIET.* For whatever reason(s), *the Stillman Diet* was known as the drinking man's diet. I guess if you liked beer and wanted to lose weight, *Stillman* was your go to diet plan. The problem with low carb diets is simple to understand: once you've experienced initial weight loss, usually in the form of water weight, as soon as car-bohydrates are again ingested, the weight returns. *The Stillman Diet* did not allow fruits or vegetables. Nor did it allow fiber which could easily lead to constipation. It burdened the kidneys and could cause ketoacidosis, a serious condition that can lead to diabetic coma, passing out for long periods of time and even death. As a quick aside, I've know friends who have sworn by the *Atkins Diet.* They have passed out in my presence while on *Atkins.* I make no connection, merely an observation.

There was the *1,000 Calorie Diet* that allowed you no more that 1,000 calories per day. The problem with diets of this ilk is starvation. 1,000 calories a day is not nutrition-ally sound or even healthy, especially for an adolescent. A certain number of calories per day are needed simply to keep you alive and maintain bodily functions such as breathing and digestion. Variables such as height, weight, age, gender, and level of activity dictate sound caloric intake. At the age of twelve I was on the *1,000 Calorie Diet.* I was a fairly active little girl and my caloric intake given my age, height, weight and level of activity should have been a little over 2,000 calories per day. The *1,000 Calorie Diet* was literally starving me.

Whenever one diet didn't work, Mom was always quick to find another, and an-other and another, including the *Cabbage Soup Diet.* Although not suitable for long-term weight loss, the *Cabbage Soup Diet* is a low-fat, high-fiber diet that will help you get into shape fast before you embark on a more moderate long-term eating plan. The diet claims that you can lose up to ten pounds in seven days. Since most folks are looking for a quick fix, this plan seems quite appealing. But unless you continue with a more rigorous or even moderate diet, the weight will return as quickly as it was lost. It never worked for me.

When it appeared dieting wasn't working or wasn't the answer, Mom would sup-plement the various diet plans with ingenious products like the *Relax-a-cizor.* The *Relax-a-cizor* was hailed as an exercise device that allowed exercising while relaxing.

The machine is tantamount to a medieval torture device. It was an electric muscle stimulation unit that claimed you can exercise while relaxing without effort. There was nothing really relaxing about this device at all. It employed large pads used on the thighs, buttocks, back, and abdominal wall. Small volts of electricity shocked various muscle groups causing the muscles to jump. Now there's a day at the beach. In 1971, the Food and Drug Administration warned that the sale of second hand *Relax-a-cizors* was illegal as people were attempting to dispose of the torturous Torquemada product. The FDA then sent "wanted posters" to post offices across the nation warning against the use of the *Relax-a-cizor*.

And, of course, there were the diet pills; amphetamine derivatives better known as speed. Enough said.

When it comes to weight loss, eating, or anything associated with food, my childhood memories haunt me like the ghost of Hamlet's father. One particular memory forever emblazoned in the recesses of my mind is the evening meal. Ah, dinner time with the family was always such a joyous occasion. My mother, an excellent, creative, and inventive cook, took great pride in preparing the evening repast for her family. Dinner was always served promptly at five per my father's orders. Daddy was a career military officer and very stringent about when and how the family would spend time together, especially at dinner time. We all had our place at the table with Daddy at the head, Mom to his right and me and my three younger brothers and sister seated accordingly by age. Being the oldest, I sat immediately to Daddy's left. Now, given the exactness of the families seating arrangements one might perceive that being the eldest daughter I would be served first or at least second following my father. Not so. Mom would first serve up generous portions of lasagna, meatballs, spaghetti (yes, in the 1960's pasta was known as spaghetti) to Daddy, then the boys, then my sister. She would then methodically remove my plate from in front of me and plop down a small, eight ounce can of *Metrecal*. For those not old enough to recall *Metrecal*, it was the *Slimfast* of its day: a powdery mix to which either water or skim milk was added. It came in a variety of flavors and was touted as the preferred diet drink of it's day. While the rest of my family enjoyed satiating themselves with Mom's wonderful Italian cuisine, I was left to sip through a straw the most nauseating fluid imaginable, all the while my mother bellowing *"Just another ten pounds, Betty, just another ten pounds!"* And thus my life long struggle with weight loss began.

How many times have you tried to go on a diet? Well, if you are like me, dozens of times. And of course, diets began every Monday of every week for most of my life! To paraphrase Mark Twain, *dieting is easy, I've been on thousands of them!* Yes, I've tried them all and none of them worked. Something was always missing. While I was on a low carb diet I craved fruits and vegetables. On those foods that were delivered diets I wanted to cook! On low calorie diets I wanted to die! Dieting becomes a chore, a way of life and a not very pleasant way of life at that.

It has been said that everything happens for a reason, that there is karma to life. Even the most mundane of activities can quite possibly have meaning or bring forth some sort of apocryphal message meant to change our lives forever. You may not realize it at the moment it happens, but upon reflection you recall it well. We've all had these moments. Such a moment came about for me while engaging in one of my favorite activities — clothes shopping. What girl doesn't like to shop for clothes? Well, when you are tipping the scales at around two hundred and fifty pounds, clothes shopping can be a nightmare. Not only was clothes shopping a nightmare at two hundred fifty pounds, I was terribly unhealthy. I was on all sorts of medication for high cholesterol, high blood pressure, acid reflux, sleep apnea, and chronic back pain which had me in therapy once a week. I was walking around like I was one hundred years old!. So I asked a friend to assist me in my nightmarish quest to find suitable new clothing for a cruise. She agreed. And what a frightening nightmare it was. I needed some *fancy* attire and everything in my size twenty two was just too dowdy and shapeless. It was a nightmare! After prowling through rack after rack of frumpish, formless blouses, skirts, dresses, and other sundry items, we stopped shopping for awhile to have lunch; of course we were going to eat. No activity is complete without food. At lunch, my friend said she had a serious problem and she didn't know who else to turn to or who could possibly help her. She sounded very serious. I waited with baited breath. What possible horror was my friend about to confide to me? Did she have cancer or some other equally dire health problem? Was she leaving her husband? Was something amiss with her daughter? No, it was none of the above. My friend's dilemma was this: she was a fat slob and had to lose five whole pounds. Yes, my friend told me she was a fat slob who couldn't control herself or her terrible eating habits and begged me to attend a weight loss meeting with her as this was her last chance. And you thought Custer had problems. There I sat, two hundred and fifty hulking pounds and she's lamenting about five pounds. Please, Louise! Honestly, I couldn't believe my ears. But because I was such a pushover (or so I thought at the time), I relented and promised my friend when I got back from my cruise, I would go with her to a weight loss meeting. When the day arrived for that initial meeting, I told my friend on the way in the door that as soon as she lost her five pounds I was outta there. But something happened. The facilitator of the meeting took an interest in me and I felt a connection. Slowly I started to understand the issues that were causing me to overeat. That's when change began to occur.

There is almost always a reason that we put on weight. My problem was emotional eating. Anytime anything went wrong, I would comfort myself with food. I thought to myself that I just loved food. Really? And I needed a lot of comforting. I had lost my job, then lost my sister, and then lost my only child, all in a very short period of time. I used food to stuff my feelings about these events into some emotional drawer.

I eventually realized that if I simply took baby steps, I would lose .06 pounds a week. Losing .06 pounds a week translated into thirty pounds a year. I thought this was doable and at thirty pounds a year, it would take me three years to attain my goal weight. Now, no one in their right mind would be satisfied with that idea. But I wasn't in my right mind. Or perhaps I was. The reason why I say that is losing that little amount of weight a week is infinitely easier than losing two pounds a week. I could give up 1,700 calories a week but 7,000 calories? Not a chance. It takes 3,500 calories to lose one pound.

I can't say that I was thrilled with those slow results, but here I am, 93 pounds thinner after three years and all because of losing .06 pounds per week. Patience in trying to lose weight is the most important part of this type of weight loss. It's all baby steps. *"By perseverance even the snail reached the ark."* (Quote from Charles H. Spurgeon)

CHAPTER TWO

THE STAGES OF WEIGHT LOSS

DENIAL

Usually I could come up with dozens of reason why I COULDN'T lose weight "I'm big boned, it's genetic," "my mother, father and grandparents were all over weight and struggled most of their lives with health issues associated with obesity." I, too suffered with health issues like high cholesterol, sleep apnea, acid reflux, and high blood pressure. And don't talk to me about *slow metabolism*. Slow metabolism leading to obesity and weight gain is about as rare as leprosy. Don't we always get our thyroid gland checked to make sure we don't have a thyroid problem and we are always a little disappointed when the results reveal our thyroid glands are working just fine. My personal favorite denial is, "I just love food." That's what I told myself, "I just love to eat." Well, who doesn't? There is almost always a reason we are overeating. I know that there are many reasons we are trying to soothe ourselves with food. Stress, sorrow, anger, disappointments even good times and celebrations can cause overeating. The most ironic celebration is when we actually reach our healthy weight and celebrate by going out to dinner. We think that whatever is wrong in our lives might be fixed by overeating. Its our go to remedy. I remember a story where a little boy skinned his knee and was crying. After cleaning and bandaging the wound, his mother gave him two cookies and told the boy that the cookies would make it better. After a little while the boy said the cookies didn't work. He hadn't eaten the cookies; he had placed them on his knee over the bandage. Even that little boy knew that food wasn't the answer.

I know that there are circumstances for many of us that an occasional binge is just going to happen. I have had three major binges and many small ones since I reached my goal. That is a definite success for me because most days before I started to lose weight were binge days.

Denial can last for years and years. It did with me. It doesn't have to with you.

ANGER

We are mad at ourselves. We are mad at others, especially those people who seem to be able to eat to their heart's content without ever gaining an ounce. We are mad at the world! The best example is my sister, Lori. Every time we go to dinner she orders fettuccine alfredo, the most fattening thing on most menus. And her house is like a bakery. Her pantry is filled with chips and cookies. I just couldn't understand how she could stay so trim. If I had all the stuff in my house I would eat every bit of it. So I decided I would try to eat like her and see what happened. I watched her eat the fettuccine alfredo and noticed she played with it more than she ate it. I am sure at the end of the meal she only consumed a half a cup, and she can actually eat just one cookie. It is a gift. The gift she possesses is portion control. There is nothing you "can't" eat if you have just one portion. So, at the end of the day, the fork is in our hand.

AWARENESS

Awareness is my favorite stage. I remember going to my favorite hamburger restaurant and finding out the burger I was about to eat had 1,900 calories in it. I simply could not justify eating that many calories at one meal. That is all the calories I get for a day. That's when my weight loss kicked into the idea that it was a lifestyle change and not just for now. Just writing down what you eat is an eye opener. I found many formulas that told me how many calories I needed a day to maintain my weight at two hundred fifty pounds. I had to consume approximately 3,000 calories a day in order to sustain a weight of two hundred fifty pounds. Certainly I can eat fewer calories. And that's when I came up with the "Banking Method" of weight loss that you will read about in chapter 8.

ACTION

I often hear, "I'm not in the right frame of mind to diet." I don't think there is a right frame of mind. I wasn't at all in the frame of mind either, and I think that was one of the best things that could have happened to me. I wasn't ready. When you are in the right frame of mind, you go all out doing all the right things, but you can just burn yourself out trying too hard. Believe me, I was not trying too hard, and that was what led to slow, very slow weight loss. I lost .6 pounds a week. Remember, it took me three years to lose ninety three pounds. So not being ready is a way to slowly move toward your goals rather than trying too hard. Slow change is better and important to maintenance.

The other thing I hear is I have to lose weight for a wedding or reunion or some other occasion. What happens when the occasion passes? Most of us revert back to our old ways because we have set a time limit on our goal, and now it's over. We need to lose weight for "FOREVER"!

In the beginning I would bring food with me that I could eat, but all that did was make me feel deprived, and when you deprive yourself too much of your food pleasure (pumpkin pie at Thanksgiving, cheeseburgers at barbecues) believe me, you will make up for it somewhere else.

There is one great thing that happens once you start to eat healthy — bad food makes you sick. One client related a story about her plan for an anniversary dinner. She wanted fried clams. She banked her calories for the week so she could enjoy one of her favorite meals. The next week when I saw her I asked how the clams were (a little vicarious living), and she told me she never felt so sick. I can relate to that. If I eat fried food now, it doesn't affect me very well.

The other part of this is that you have to get sick an awful lot to get back to your bad eating habits. Unfortunately, I occasionally have to be reminded to this.

SUCCESS

I think success is measured in five pound increments. They say maintenance is harder than losing the weight. If you gain five pounds after reaching your goal and you take steps to lose it, that is success.

I have played many times with those five pounds; too many times. I think you should always have five pounds to lose, not that you shouldn't be satisfied but more to keep in check because five pounds can lead to ten pounds and before you know it, you are back where you started x amount of pounds ago.

So success is all about five pounds.

INTANGIBLE SUCCESSES

Sometime, somewhere, someone once proclaimed, *I never said it was going to be easy, I said it would be worth it.* And so it has been with the struggles I've experienced with weight loss, keeping unwanted pounds off and maintaining a healthy life style. It hasn't been easy; dear lord it hasn't been easy but I must say, it has been worth it. Once the pounds have been shed, a whole new world view dramatically opens up in so many ways. One of my first experiences with a new found world view, post weight loss was clothes shopping. For years I sought a simple, cute denim jean jacket to wear on those cool summer evenings when a sweater just didn't make the grade. Being a robust 250 pound girl, it was difficult to find such a jacket. Once I had lost the 93 pounds, new worlds of shopping opportunities opened up to me. I was shopping for the jacket, rifling through racks of what I thought were sizes I should be looking at when a sales lady approached me and said, "You shouldn't be looking here, you want the other side of the store, dear." Now in days gone by, I probably would have been slightly insulted by a salesperson who was attempting to herd me to the plus size section of the store - the other side of the store. But now, the salesperson was sending me from the plus side of the store to the under size 18 side of the store - hallowed ground I had heretofore never ventured. I was never more happy in my life; I was shopping on the other side of the store.

CHAPTER THREE

THE ROAD TO HELL-TH

The road to hell-th is paved with good intentions. You know how it is. Every Sunday evening when you go to bed, full from eating all day, bloated, uncomfortable, guilty, you say to yourself, "tomorrow I'm going to be good, I'm going to do everything right or what I perceive to be right." Unfortunately for most people, what they perceive to be right is an all or nothing proposition. Every Monday doesn't have to be a New Year's Resolution. Don't set yourself up for failure. Don't believe you are going to begin an exercise regiment by walking three miles the first day, by doing one hundred sit ups or by denying yourself food. If you do, you're going to start writing exercise checks that by Wednesday your body won't be able to cash. Let's face it, you probably haven't been to a gym or worked out in a month of Sundays, and your body just isn't ready for that kind of rigorous work out. You'll become frustrated, discouraged, and will soon give up. Yes, the road to hell-th is paved with good intentions. Make those intentions doable.

So here's the question: what's between *all* or *nothing*? It's got to be something, right? What's your priority, what's most important? Do you want to lose the weight or do you want to keep it off? The something in between *all* and *nothing* can be small, incremental baby steps; steps that you can manage, steps that will help you begin to understand you can accomplish goals. It doesn't have to be *all* or *nothing*.

QUESTIONS

Here are some questions you should ask yourself: Can I walk for twenty minutes? Can I eat salad at one meal each day of the week? Can I make sure I had a healthy breakfast? The cumulative effect of all these little things that aren't too, too hard will begin to pay dividends over time. Perseverance. This is what I believe is so hard about dieting. We try to get to a goal as fast as humanly possible without thinking of what is going to happen once we get there. You cannot lose weight one way and keep it off another.

BREAKING DOWN THE BABY STEPS

What weight loss goal is right for you? Remember, it's baby steps so the goals should initially be short term. Here are a few suggestions for you to do weekly in order to set you on the road to a healthy lifestyle editing process.

1. The first step in setting a goal for weight loss is to remember to accentuate the positive, to keep and remain upbeat. Don't minimize your accomplishments by saying things like "*I only lost_____ pounds.*" Lose the weight and lose the word *only*! I don't care if you lost two grams, you lost weight, you didn't gain weight! Be affirmative about your accomplishments.

2. If you decide to exercise, start slowly. On the first day walk a half mile. Don't over do it. Be happy and content you walked the half mile. When that half mile starts to become easier, add a quarter mile and so forth an so on. You'll be surprised at how quickly you'll soon be walking three miles.

3. On Monday make sure you drink a minimum of forty-eight ounces of water. Often times when we think we're hungry, water will satisfy those cravings. Water is a great diarrhetic. It keeps you hydrated and for those of us who eat out of some sort of oral compulsion, drinking water assumes that role. Most importantly, *write down everything you eat.*

4. On Tuesday make sure you eat fruits and vegetables. Most importantly, *write down everything you eat.*

5. On Wednesday make sure you exercise, eat lean protein, and *write down everything you eat.*

6. On Thursday eat more fruits and vegetables, and *write down everything you eat.*

7. On Friday exercise again and drink a minimum of forty eight ounces of water, and *write down everything you eat.*

8. On Saturday take some time and plan what you are going to eat for the week so you're prepared and *write down everything you eat.*

9. On Sunday, rest.

You have to figure out how you can lose weight slowly and be able to handle it. Here's where the perseverance plays a major role. When I lost weight, I can tell you in all honesty, I wasn't patient at all. I did lose 30 pounds a year and that was 93 pounds in the end but it took me three years. It took me three years because I was a cheater, a bad cheater! I couldn't have just one cookie, I had to have six cookies! If I like a particular food, I'd eat it to death or to the point of being uncomfortable! I never counted calories on the weekends. And I would drink Espresso martinis! I still cheat. and when I do, later that day or the next day, I'll get a food hangover, because my body is not use to the sugar or lard I've consumed. And because I exercise, I know I'll have to walk miles to work off all that sugar! It's just not worth it. Whatever you eat has to be calorie worthy.

As a result of all my cheating, I would actually lose very little weight and be shocked and surprised by this phenomenon every time. I would always act like I should have lost at least three pounds when in fact I gained two. My indignation was profound. But who was I really kidding? I wasn't doing what I needed to do in order to lose the kind of weight I wanted to lose. Then I began to realize that I could still lose the weight even if it was a slow process. I started to build on that. Lose a little, hold it. Lose a little bit more, hold it. I was beginning to understand that this perseverance, these slow and steady baby steps would work for me. I realized that the only way I could lose weight was slowly; .06 pounds a week was the best I could do. I wasn't about to break any weight loss records, but I was steadily losing and not gaining back two pounds for every three I lost.

Now just imagine yourself thirty pounds lighter exactly one year from now. That would be so unbelievable! Who wouldn't take that kind of loss? So on Monday, why don't you try simply do to a few little things, and on Tuesday a few more different little things, and as we go through it together, I'll give you some ideas on how to take those little baby steps. Because really, that's what you have to do. It's all baby steps. The truth is, we only want to lose this weight once. Isn't once torture enough? Think of the numerous diets you've tried. If we do it slowly we have every chance of keeping the weight off, because we are changing our life style or we are editing our life style. So motivation doesn't last. Think about this: on the cover of every weight loss magazine is the same old promise of losing twenty pounds in twenty days by eating this fruit or that protein or this candy bar or this health drink. We all know none of it's true, so why do we want to be fooled? Are we really gluttons for diet punishment? Here's the deal: we want quick results but even if you lost twenty pounds in twenty days you're probably just going to gain all that weight back and then some. You can't lose weight one way and keep it off another. Don't diet, *EDIT*.

The road to hell-th is a long and winding one. It meanders, curves, serves up potholes and other obstacles, sometimes limits our speed but often offers exits to highways of success. In January of 2011 I widened that road to hell-th with the formation of my own company, *Losing Weight With Elizabeth*, a practical and permanent way to lose weight, keep weight off and maintain a healthy life style. *Losing Weight With Elizabeth* provides the support of small group meetings coupled with a customized program to meet individual goals. Our members enjoy a one to one orientation to the program and are provided with ongoing connections to weight loss resources. We help members learn to create individualized eating plans, food shopping and introduce them to the "banking" method of weight loss which you'll read more about in chapter 8.

If indeed the road to hell-th is paved with good intentions, one particular intention near and dear to is to share

CHAPTER FOUR

HEALTHY HABITS

The road to losing that .06 pounds per week is filled with additional pothole like challenges, challenges that come in the form of behavior modifications, also known as tricks you play on yourself to change your eating habits. It's been said to me on more than one occasion that I should put my fork down between bites of food in order to slow down the "inhaling" process. I never seemed to be able to follow that particular rule, so I modified the modifier and came up with my own method: "never put food in your mouth when you have food in your mouth." For those of us who love to shovel food or inhale food, and I was one, this simple mantra was a great baby step on my road to success. I did indeed slow down my eating process and realized when I was satisfied.

I always knew I had bad posture. I was 5' 7" tall in the 8th grade, towering over most boys in my class, over weight, and slouching. The slouching became habitual and carried on into adulthood. One day while driving and becoming annoyed with the number of traffic lights I was stopping at, I had a bit of an epiphany. What if, every time I came to a traffic light that was red I held in my stomach until it turned green? Why not? What could it hurt? It gave me something to do at red lights and might help improve my posture. It's been said if you stand up straight and hold your stomach in, you look ten pounds thinner. Who doesn't want to look ten pounds thinner? Here's the operative question: how did this help in my weight loss? Well, I became much more aware of my posture by employing this baby step modifier of holding my stomach in at traffic lights and eventually found myself using it throughout the day. This baby step is very effective.

I love to cook. One draw back to overweight people cooking is their penchant for sampling; eating while cooking. I would often eat an entire meal while preparing the meal! I would eat the meal twice, once while preparing it and then again when I sat down with my husband or guests. I needed to change this habit quickly so I decided I would never put food in my mouth while standing. That should work, right? You're in the kitchen preparing a meal and on your feet so if you're standing, and adhering to a rule about not eating unless you're seated, you should be okay. I challenged myself by putting a chair in the kitchen while preparing meals and immediately became aware of how many times I would sit down during meal preparation. I must have sat down at least ten times. The key here was self awareness and being able to recognize the need to change behavior. I realized every bad habit I possessed was going to take some serious but reasonable and easy ways to address. I had to get creative. Taking these few baby steps pushed me in the right direction and made me much more aware.

TREAT YOURSELF LIKE COMPANY

Let's face it, we love to eat. So why is it that we eat standing up or in the car or anywhere that is not really conducive to enjoying our food. So I say treat yourself like you would company.

1. Use a table cloth and cloth napkins (go green without paper).
2. Drink from a fancy glass.
3. Use smaller plates and bowls.
4. Flowers if possible.
5. Candles.
6. Involve others.
7. Try new foods.
8. Have a few courses. A salad or soup will fill you up so you aren't apt to eat too much.

One of my members used this idea with her daughter one night. They didn't have fresh flowers so they used plastic ones and they didn't have candles so they used their "emergency" one. The daughter was so happy to have a "fancy" dinner that she took it upon herself to make sure the table looked nice every time she and her mother sat down for a meal. It is just nice.

RESTAURANT RULES

1. If you can, choose the restaurant that you know you can have some food you like and not feel deprived. If you can choose the restaurant, and you know that you are going to be tested with too many temptations, eat as healthy and low calories as you can that day.

2. Know what you are going to have before you go. Lots of restaurants have their menus online and some have the calories. Plan for it.

3. Don't go hungry. You'll ruin your dinner eating the entire bread basket!

4. Don't listen to the specials. The second I hear the words "infused with," "cream," or Bearnaise, all bets are off.

5. Make sure whatever you are eating is calorie worthy.

6. Eat slowly and enjoy yourself. You will find that you are full faster.

7. Three ways to save calories: share a meal, have the server pack one-half of your dinner, have soup and salad or appetizer and salad.

8. If you are having alcoholic drinks, have a glass of water between drinks.

9. Share a desert. This is always a good plan. A piece of cheesecake can be over five hundred calories.

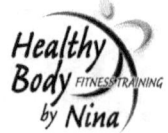

CHAPTER FIVE

HEALTHY BODY BY NINA

SQUATS – Stand with feet about hip width apart, dumbbells by the side of your body. Put your weight on your heels and lower your buttocks as if you are going to sit down in a chair. Do not go beyond 90 degrees of your knees. Push through your heels to come back up to starting position. **Harder** – Add an overhead press when coming back to starting position.

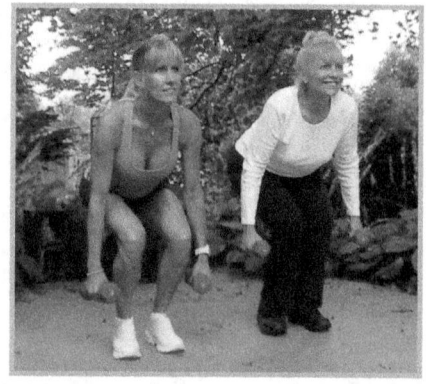

PLIE SQUAT – Stand with feet wide apart, toes slightly angled out, dumbbells by the side. Lower your buttocks straight down (think of having a glass of water to balance on top of your head without spilling). Do not go beyond 90 degrees of your knees. Squeeze your glutes when you push back up to starting position. **Harder** – Add lateral raises. Lift dumbbells out to the side no higher than shoulder height when you come back to starting position.

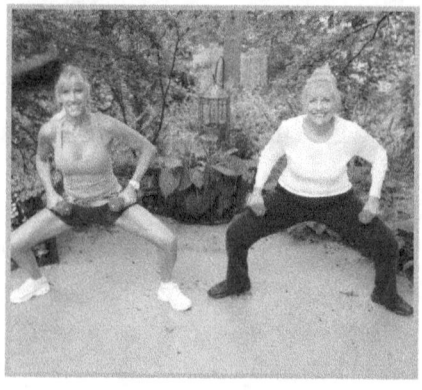

DEAD LIFTS –

Stand with dumbbells in front of your thighs, fold from the hips (make sure to keep your back flat) let the hamstring stretch and then activate hamstrings and glutes to come back to starting position. **Harder** – One leg extends.

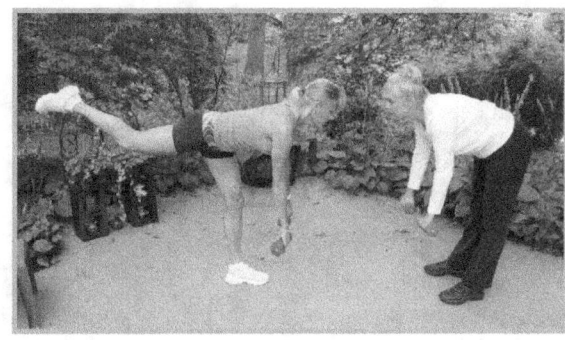

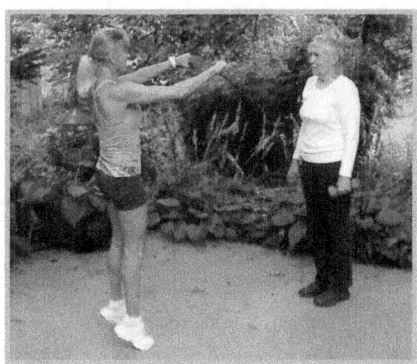

HEEL RAISES – Stand with feet comfortable distance apart. The closer the harder. Rise up on the ball of your feet with stable ankles. Lower to starting position. **Harder** – Add front raises

CHEST PRESS

– In supine position with dumbbells by your chest, palms facing your thighs. Press dumbbells up chest width apart and slowly lower them back to chest.

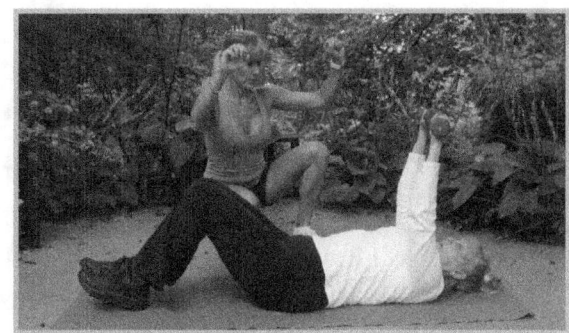

Harder – Add bridge when you press dumbbells up.

CHEST FLIES –

In supine position start with dumbbells straight over chest palms facing each other, elbows slightly bent. Slowly let the arms out to the sides like butterfly wings.

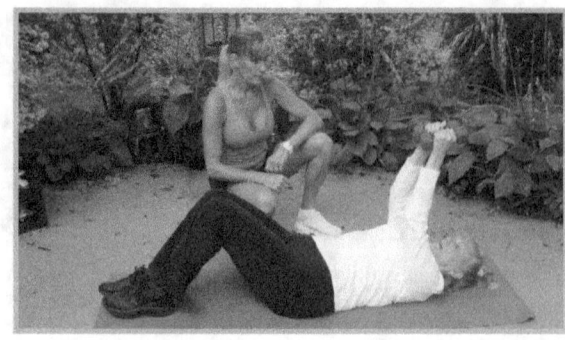

Squeeze your pecs to bring them back to starting position. **Harder** – Alternating one arm at the time.

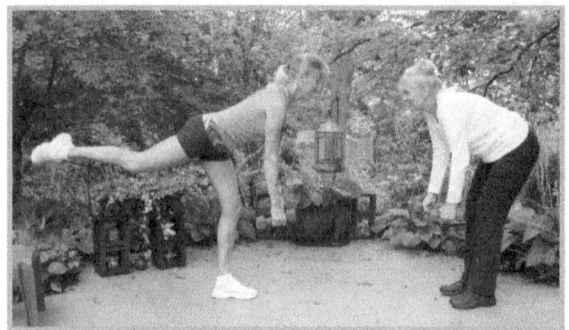

BENT-OVER-ROW

– Fold by the hips, make sure back is flat, and engage your abdominals to protect your back. Pull the dumbbells up to your waist; squeeze your shoulder blades together. **Harder** – Keep one leg extended and switch after half of the repetitions.

BICEPS CURLS WITH A TWIST

– Bring dumbbells up towards your shoulders with a twist. Keep elbows by waistline.
Harder – Alternating lunges.

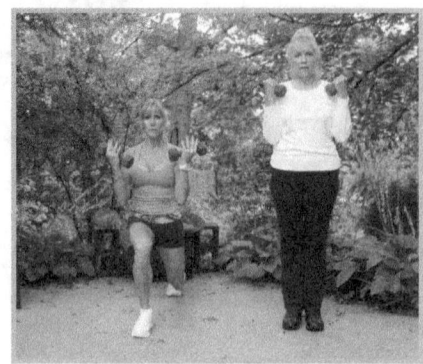

TRICEPS KICKBACKS –

Fold from hips, elbows high and close to body, hands by the waist, press dumbbells back all the way. Elbows stay stationary as you extend them.

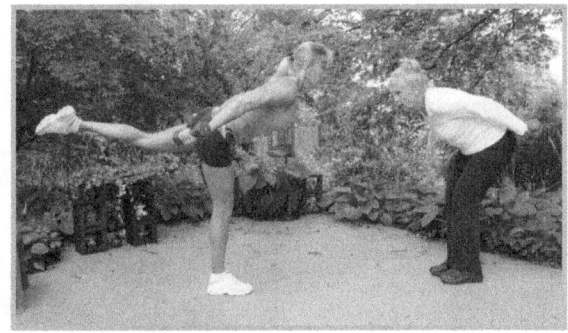

Harder – Balance on one leg and switch after half of the reps.

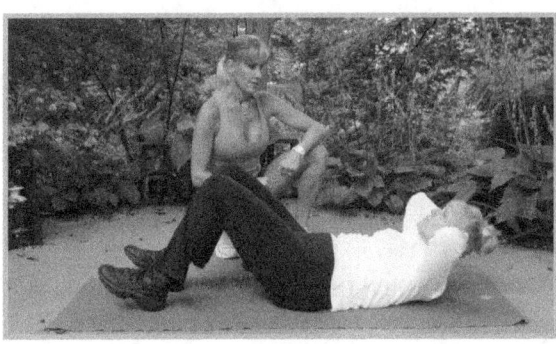

STRAIGHT CRUNCHES –

In supine position, pull your navel towards the spine and lift shoulder blades off the floor. Think of bringing the ribcage towards your hip-bones. Keep the distance open between your chin and your chest. **Harder** – bring your knees to chest as you crunch and extend them when you lower the shoulder blades.

CROSS OVER CRUNCHES –

In supine position bring right shoulder towards left knee and then left shoulder to-wards right knee. Do not pull the elbow to-

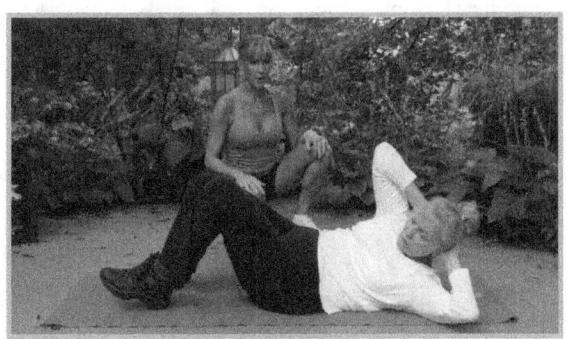

wards the knee, think of ribcage contracting towards opposite hipbone to engage the oblique. **Harder** – Bicycle crunches, alternating shoulder to opposite knee.

SUPERMAN –

In prone position, hands by shoulders lift your chest up from floor engaging the muscle that goes along the spine. **Harder** – extend arms in front of your body and lift arms and legs simultaneously.

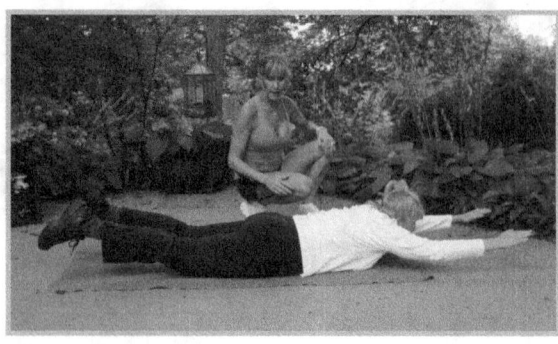

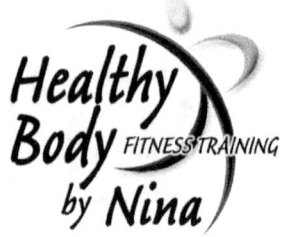

Nina Lane was born and raised in Sweden. She lived an active lifestyle participating in various sports growing up. At age 15 Nina played on an adult volleyball team that was number 2 in Sweden at the time. She always had an interest for languages as well and studied English, French, and Spanish.

1988 Nina decided to come to United States to improve her English. She ended up working as a linguist at a linguistic software company. She competed in triathlons and running. Her interest for sports and fitness naturally led her in to the fitness industry where she started as a group instructor a few nights a week after her linguist job. 3 years later she gave up her linguist job and focused on the fitness job. Nina was soon promoted as the fitness director for our YMCA where she worked for 14 years before starting her own fitness studio focusing on one-on-one training. Each year the number of clients increased and now she has 3 certified personal trainers working with her. Nina is a certified personal trainer, group fitness instructor, mat Pilates, Pilates reformer trainer, and cycling instructor. Her fitness studio is Healthy Body by Nina located on Marco Island, Florida.

Nina is the loving mother of two teenagers. Patrick whom is eighteen and attends Lewis & Clark College in Portland, Or. and Alessea age of sixteen and is an Honors student at Lely High School.

CHAPTER SIX

MEAL PLANNING

The following are diaries from real people
living the Banking Method

1300 calories a day

Breakfast
1 c. water + 6 ice cubes+1/2 tsp of vanilla
1 c. fresh blueberries
1 tbs. paleo fibre-
½ container of light and fit vanilla yogurt

162 cal

Lunch
1 oz. cooked diced chicken
2 c. salad
2 tbs. of balsamic vinegar
2 baby carrots, celery, green & red pepper   138 cal

snack
1 beer Corona
1 diet coke
H.M. blueberry & strawberry pie w/cool whip   279 cal
¼ c. Yogurt ice cream   75 cal
1 Milano cookie   110 cal

Dinner
1 ½ . c. of pasta   275 cal
1/3 c . sauce   90 cal
Salad: cucumbers, lettuce,red peppers, parsley   10 Cal

Total 1,139 calories
....

7/21/11
Breakfast
1 hard boiled egg   2inch x 2" piece of Portuguese bread   210 calories

lunch
vegetable tortellini soup + half of a peach   230 Calories

snack
Popcorn   400 calories
Diet soda

Dinner
Spinach, strawberry salad, chicken, w/dressing   335 calories
1 glass cabernet sauvinguion wine   87 cal

total 1212 calories
****

7/22/11
Breakfast
½ c.cherrios, lactaid free milk, fruit nut granola
tea w/ lemon   240 calories

Lunch
H. M Tortellini soup with vegetables +tea w/lemon   230 calories

Dinner
Four raviolis + sauce
1 piece of vegetable pizza with sausage
Salad: lettuce, tomato, radishes, cucumber (balsamic vinegar)
1 large glass red wine
1inch X 2 inch brownie with nuts   785 calories

total 1,255 calories

7/23/11 Saturday

Breakfast
H.M. blueberry pie +1/2 small grapefruit + tea w/lemon   302 calories

Lunch
3 raviolis with sauce + iced tea w/ lemon   330 cal

(forgot to write it down)

7/24/11 Sunday
Breakfast
1 egg + catsup on a wheat round, toasted w/ hot tea   176 calories

Lunch
1 piece of pizza with veggies w/iced tea w/ lemon   332 calories

Dinner
Turkey burger, 4 oz on a wheat roll w/ catsup +salad*   250 calories

Total 768 calories
****

7/25/11 Monday
Breakfast
½ S.B. cinnamon scone; 6 cherries, 1 slice watermelon + hot tea   442 calories

Lunch
Salad: lettuce, cucumber, radishes, tomato, (balsamic vinegar) + 5 club
crackers   105 Calories

Dinner
6 inch veggie delight; wheat subway w/ oil and vinegar + diet coke   280 calories

Total 827 Calories
....
*All salads are topped with balsamic vinegar only
unless stated otherwise; H.M. = home made; S.B. Store bought

28

Lynn ☺

Breakfast 🐾

Egg + Asparagus Omelet
    2 eggs + 2 tsp of fat   250 🐾
    1/2 cup of Asparagus   + 20
                        270
    1/2 cup of mango slices   + 55 🐾
                        325

Snack 🐾
Emerald's Breakfast-on-the-Go   + 180
   1 Pouch   505 🐾

Lunch
Regular Salad   10 🐾
Top with 2oz of Kirland's Wild
Sockeye Salmon   60
Newman's Own - Light Balsamic 🐾
  Vinaigrette   45
                      115 🐾

Snack
Snyder's Dipping Pretzels (count 14)   120
Artichoke + Olive Hummus (2 tbsp)   60 🐾
                      180

Dinner 🐾
Pork Tenderloin (4oz)   250
Mashed Sweet Potato (1/2 cup)   125
Tomato (1 med-sliced) + Cucumber (1/2 cup)   35 🐾
Light Italian Dressing (2 Tbsp)   65
                      575
Dessert Pudding Snack @   total = 1475 🐾
    100 calories

1500 calorie day

Breakfast
- Fiber One Thin Sandwich Roll — 90 cal.
- 1 Hard Boiled Egg (Sliced) — 105 cal.
- 1 Large slice of Tomato — N/A cal.
- Spread ½ of Light Laughing Cow Cheese — 17 cal.
- 1 cup of any 50 cal. diet juice — 50 cal.

total 262 cal.

Snack
- Any 100 calorie yogurt — 100 cal.

total 362 cal.

Lunch
- See Any one of the "American Pie" choices (300 cal. or less) — 300 cal.

total 662 cal.

Snack
- 1 medium apple — 70 cal.
- 2 tbsp of peanut butter — 190 cal.

total 922 cal.

Dinner
- 3 oz of Flank Steak (broiled or grilled) — 155 cal
- Baked Sweet Potato with 1 tbsp butter — 90 cal. / 100 cal.
- String Beans (Steamed) 4 oz. with Almonds (24-28) — 40 cal. / 170 cal.

total 1477 cal.

*Skip afternoon snack, and have snack at night. ≈ 300 calories.

Breakfast   Lynn   calories 🐾
   2 hard-boiled eggs   130
   Quick oatmeal (fix according to pkg)   150
   cinnamon - 6 tsp, blueberries - 15   31
   splenda - 0, vanilla - 10 tsp   +
     311 🐾

Snack Chobani Cherry Yogurt   +140
     451 🐾

Lunch
   2 cups of Progresso   +160
   Chicken Barley Soup   611 🐾

Snack   11 Kirland Chocolate Covered   +160 🐾
     Almonds   771

Dinner   This serves 2 people!! 🐾
Stir-fry Chicken (4oz - lightly floured)   280
Use Pam spray   6 🐾
Peppers - 30 1 med., Tomato - 25 1 med.   ½ of = 515
   (both diced)
Marinated Artichoke Hearts (2oz.)   50 🐾
All over Barilla (4oz.) Cut Spaghetti   400

Dessert 🐾
   Friendly's Vienna Mocha Swirl   300
     1 cup 🐾

Beverages during the day
are water, diet soda or   total = 1466 !! 🐾
Life water = 0   for the day

31

Breakfast
Fiber One Thin Sandwich   Lynn
Roll (whole Grain white)   90 calories
Spread : 1 tblsp of peanut butter   95
          1 tblsp of grape jelly   50
          1/2 small banana (sliced)   45
                                          280

Lunch
Shrimp + Asparagus - recipe
1 lb of Asparagus (steamed + cut)
1 lb of medium shrimp
1 cup of grape tomatoes (cut in half)
1/2 thinly sliced onion (optional)
2 tblsp chopped parseley
2 hard boiled eggs (sliced
season with salt, pepper & 1 1/2 tblsps olive
oil
  2 tbsps of lemon juice
  serving size 1 1/2 cups =   225

Dinner
  Angel hair pasta (4 ounces)
6 medium Roma tomatoes (chopped)
1/4 cup chopped fresh basil
2 tblsps of light butter, 1 tsp of garlic (chopped)
Shredded Parmesan cheese
Cook pasta as usual. In large
skillet cook over medium heat (1-2 mins.)
Toss pasta together with tomato mixture →

in a large serving bowl.
2 cup serving   400

280 + 225 + 400 =   905

I usually snack on Chabani Yogurt
in the morning — 140 cal!   1045 cal

If you are consuming 1500
calories ... you can have a
dessert at night after dinner of
400 calories! (That's usually a cup
of ice cream for me !!!)

(Breakfast)   Lynn

3/4 cup Quaker Oats
Quick – 1 min. Oatmeal   225 cal.
fix according to pkg. with H₂O
Add in: 1/2 tsp of Vanilla
        1/2 tsp of cinnamon
        1 beaten egg (raw →   75
        stir into cooked oatmeal)
Chop and add 1/2 of small apple   27
            1/2 of small banana   45   or
            1/2 cup of blueberries   15   or
            1/2 cup of strawberries   25
        Total cal 327 or 345 or 315 or 325
note: to sweeten add Splenda (1 packette) 0

(Snack) (before or after lunch)
Chobani Cherry Yogurt   140

(Lunch)
Fiber One Thin Sandwich Roll   90
  (Whole Grain White)
Ham (Kirkland 98% Fat Free)
  3 slices   25 cal ea   75
1 slice of tomato, 2 slices of
pickles (Stackers), Lettuce
Spread hummus or Laughing Cow
Light Cheese   35
  Huge sandwich only ——→   200

        345 + 140 + 200 = 685 ——→

Dinner
  Sockeye Salmon Fillet (4oz.)   190
  (Berkley + Jensen frozen)
  Sweet Potato (1 medium) mashed   125
  3 Bean salad (½ cup)(any deli)   110
                                     ‾‾‾‾‾
                                      425
        total after dinner   1110 cal

Dessert
Eddy's Frozen Yogurt (1cup)   220

        total calories = 1330

Breakfast

Denver Omelette in a Mug

   Recipe: 1/4 cup green bell pepper
             2 Tablespoons chopped onion
             1/2 cup fat-free liquid egg substitute
             1 ounce (about 2 slices) 97% fat free ham, chopped
             2 Tablespoons shredded fat free cheddar cheese

Spray a large microwave-safe mug with nonstick spray. Add veggies and microwave 1 to 2 minutes, until softened. Add egg substitute, mix well, microwave for 1 minute. Add ham and cheese and lightly stir. Microwave for 1 minute. Makes one serving.
122 calories

Snack

Greek yogurt   160 calories
1 cup raspberries 50 calories

Lunch

Thanksgiving in a Salad Bowl

   Recipe: 2 cups chopped romaine lettuce
             2 cups chopped spinach
             3 ounces cooked and chopped skinless lean turkey breast
             2 Tablespoons dried cranberries, chopped
             2 Tablespoons crumbled fat free feta cheese
             1 Tablespoon chopped pecans

Dressing: 1 Tablespoon canned whole cranberry sauce
            1/2 Tablespoon balsamic vinegar
            1/2 teaspoon honey mustard
            Dash salt & pepper
Makes one serving. 296 calories.

Snack

1 1/2 cups grapes   90 calories

Dinner

3 ounce ground beef patty
1 ounce cheddar cheese
light hamburger roll
2 Tablespoons BBQ sauce
470 calories

Snack

90 calorie Fiber one Bar

Total Day's Calories   1278

DELORES					
BREAKFAST	1500		BREAKFAST		1500
2-WAFFLES - 170 - 1330			2-EGGS	148 -	1352
1/3 cup Lactaid milk - 30 - 1300			2-Sl. Toast	100 -	1252
1-tsp Lacaid Butter - 15 - 1285			3-Sl. Bacon	60 -	1192
1/4- Cup Syrup - 100 - 1185			Tea/ Lacaid 1/3 milk cup 30 -		1162
LUNCH.			2-tsp Lacaid Butter 30 -		1132
1-Bowl CK.Soup - 140 - 1045			SNACK		
1/2 Panera Sand - 300 - 745			1-Choc. Bar - 210 - 922		
Water - o - ---			1-8oz. Gatorade - 50 - 872		
1-Carton O.J. 110 - 635			LUNCH		
DINNER			1-Cup CK. Soup - 180 - 692		
1- Turkey Burger - 170 - 465			15- Special R-Crackers - 61 - 631		
3 oz. Tomatoe - 15 - 450			DINNER		
10-Green Olives - 50 - 400			3-Turkey Meatballs - 140 - 491		
1-Cup Lettuce - 6 - 394			3/4 Cup Pasta - 190 - 301		
1-4 oz. Red Potatoe - 84 - 310			1/4 Cup Sauce - 20 - 281		
1-tsp. Lacaid Butter - 15 - 295			1-TBS Lacaid Butter - 45 236		
1- Sl. White Cheese - 56 - 239			SNACK		
Water - o -			2-Sl. Bread - 100 - 136		
SNACK			1-TBS. Jam - 50 - 86		
1- 100 CAL Snack - 100 - 139			Tea/ 1/3cup Lactaid milk - 30 56		
1-Special K Bar - 90 - 49			1/2 mini Coffee Cake 100 CAL. 50 - (6)		
1-Cup Tea/ Lactaid milk - 30 (19)					

1 fried egg 105
½ pat butter 17
½c OS 50
1 rye toast 80
½ pat butter 17

McDonalds wrap
  Honey Mustard Chicken ... 260
1 Magnum Ice Cream bar 240
1 sausage patty 290
  peppers & onions 30
1 c watermelon .... <u>100</u>
                        1,159

100 cal. pack .... <u>100</u>
                        1,259

Jeanne

1c oat meal	150
1/2 pat butter	17
1 plum	100
beef hot dog & roll	400
IHOP	
2 eggs - 2 bacon - 2 pancakes	670
	1337

Janie

1	egg-muffin	125
	w/ peppers - onions cheese	75
3/4c	OJ	80
1 c	strawberries	50
1 c	clam chowder	240
1 oz	oyster crackers	60
	chicken-marsala	145
	weight watcher recipe	
1/4c	small peas	30
1 c	linguine	200
2"	brownie	175
		1210

BREAKfast   1500
1-Cup tea/ 1/3 cup milk   —   30 -   1470
1-Pkg. Oatmeal Maple+ Brown Sugar —   120 -   1350
2-Slices White Toast   —   140 -   1210
1-TBS. Butter   —   45 -   1165

Lunch
1- 5oz can Tuna in water   —   100 -   1065
2-Slices Smart Bread   —   100 -   965
1-Cup Romaine Lettuce   —   6 -   959
1.5oz Tomatoe   —   8 -   951
5-Green Olives   —   25 -   926
1- 100 Cal. Snack   —   100 -   826
1-Special K-Bar   —   90 -   736
Water —

Dinner
2- Pcs. Baked Chicken 4.6 oz —   216 -   520
1 1/2 Cups Broccoli   —   45 -   475
1-TBS. Butter   —   45 -   430
1-Cup Chicken Flavor Rice   —   200 -   230
Water
Snack
1- Cup Yoplait Yogurt   —   100   130
1- 100 Cal. Snack   —   100   30
1- Clementine   —   30   —0—

Breakfast			1500
2-Low Fat Waffles	—	170	1330
3-Fat Free Sausage Links	—	190	1140
1-tsp. Lactaid Butter	—	15	1125
1-Cup tea/ 1/3 cup milk	—	30	1095

Lunch			
1-Bowl Chicken Soup	—	140	955
1/2 Panera Turkey Sand.	—	300	655
1-Carton O. J.	—	110	545

Dinner			
2-Lean Pork Chops	—	166	379
1-Sm. Baked Red Potatoe	—	145	234
1-TBS. Lactaid Butter	—	45	189
1-Cup String Beans	—	40	149

Snack			
1- 100 Calorie Coffee Cake	—	100	49
1- Cup tea/ 1/3 cup Lactaid milk	—	30	19

<u>Breakfast</u>

Egg Sandwich:

1 egg
1 slice Fat Free cheese
1 slice deli ham
on light english muffin
250 calories

<u>Snack</u>

Plain Greek yogurt 100 calories
with packet drink mix (like Crystal Light) mixed in 5 calories

<u>Lunch</u>

2 97% fat free hot dogs
2 light hot dog rolls
240 calories

<u>Snack</u>

1/4 cup trail mix 140 calories

<u>Dinner</u>

1 medium size baked potato
1 ear corn
BBQ chicken breast
spray butter
425 calories

<u>Snack</u>

1 cup blueberries 80 calories

Total Day's Calories   1240

Bill

	Bill	200.00				
7/28/2011						
Thursday	5 Cups of Coffee	25.00				
Lunch	Pita	60.00				
	Lettuces	7.00				
	Olives	36.00				
	Red Pepper	30.00				
	Broccoli	30.00				
	Cauliflower	30.00				
	Hard Cheese	220.00				
Dinner	Lettuces	7.00				
	Olives	36.00				
	Red Pepper	30.00				
	Broccoli	30.00				
	Cheese balls	100.00				
	Cauliflower	30.00				
	Dressing	60.00				
	Chicken	290.00				
	Yellow Squash	15.00				
	Zucchini	15.00				
	Jell-O	5.00				
	Yogurt	90.00				
7/29/2011						
Friday	5 Cups of Coffee	25.00				
Lunch	Pita	60.00				
	Lettuces	7.00				
	Olives	36.00				
	Red Pepper	30.00				
	Broccoli	30.00				
	Cauliflower	30.00				
	Hard Cheese	220.00				
Dinner	Lettuces	7.00				
	Olives	36.00				
	Red Pepper	30.00				
	Broccoli	30.00				
	Cheese balls	100.00				
	Cauliflower	30.00				
	Dressing	60.00				
	Turkey Burger	280.00				
	Asparagus	30.00				
	Jell-O	5.00				
	Yogurt	90.00				
7/30/2011	5 Cups of Coffee	25.00				
Saturday						

Bill

		Bill				
	Wendy's Chicken Sandwich	350.00				
	Fries	410.00				
	DD chocolate muffin	650.00				
7/31/2011	5 Cups of Coffee	25.00				
Sunday						
	Quiz no's Turkey Melt	1220.00				
	French Fries	410.00				
	Ice Cream	700.00				
8/1/2011	5 Cups of Coffee	25.00				
Monday						
Lunch	Pita	60.00				
	Lettuces	7.00				
	Olives	36.00				
	Red Pepper	30.00				
	Broccoli	30.00				
	Cauliflower	30.00				
	Hard Cheese	340.00				
	Cherries	130.00				
	Fresh Pineapple	75.00				
Dinner	Lettuces	7.00				
	Olives	36.00				
	Red Pepper	30.00				
	Broccoli	30.00				
	Cheese balls	100.00				
	Cauliflower	30.00				
	Dressing	60.00				
	Fish	275.00				
	Crab	35.00				
	Ritz Crackers	35.00				
	Butter	40.00				
	Asparagus	15.00				
	Fresh Pineapple	75.00				
8/2/2011	5 Cups of Coffee	25.00				
Tuesday						
Lunch	Pita	60.00				
	Lettuces	7.00				
	Olives	36.00				
	Red Pepper	30.00				
	Broccoli	30.00				
	Cauliflower	30.00				
	Hard Cheese	340.00				
	Cherries	130.00				
Dinner	Lettuces	7.00				
	Olives	36.00				
	Red Pepper	30.00				
	Broccoli	30.00				
	Cheese balls	100.00				

Bill

	Cauliflower	30.00				
	Dressing	60.00				
	Salmon Burger	170.00				
	String Beans	40.00				
	Jell-O	5.00				
	Yogurt	90.00				
	Cake	225.00				
8/3/2011	5 Cups of Coffee	25.00				
Wednesday						
Lunch	Pita	60.00				
	Lettuces	7.00				
	Olives	36.00				
	Red Pepper	30.00				
	Broccoli	30.00				
	Cauliflower	30.00				
	Hard Cheese	220.00				
	Cherries	130.00				
	Yogurt	100.00				
Dinner	Lettuces	7.00				
	Olives	36.00				
	Red Pepper	30.00				
	Broccoli	30.00				
	Cheese balls	100.00				
	Cauliflower	30.00				
	Dressing	60.00				
	Turkey Burger	280.00				
	Yellow Squash	15.00				
	Zucchini	15.00				
	Jell-O and Yogurt (2)	210.00				
	Cherrys	100.00				
8/4/2011	5 Cups of Coffee	25.00				
Thursday						
Lunch	Pita	60.00				
	Lettuces	7.00				
	Olives	36.00				
	Red Pepper	30.00				
	Broccoli	30.00				
	Cauliflower	30.00				
	Hard Cheese	220.00				
	Cherries	130.00				
			2000.00			
	Total for the week	11263.00	1220.00			
			780.00			

Printable Diary for **Mimioriginals**

| From: | August | 7 | 2011 | **Show:** | Food Diary | Food Notes | CHANGE REPORT |
| To: | August | 7 | 2011 | | Exercise Diary | Exercise notes | |

August 7, 2011

FOODS	Calories	Carbs	Fat	Protein	Cholest	Sodium	Sugars	Fiber
Breakfast								
Polaner All Fruit - Seedless Raspberry, 1 tablespoon	40	10g	0g	0g	0mg	0mg	9g	0g
Generic Fat Free Milk - Non-Fat Milk , 4 oz	45	7g	0g	4g	1mg	63mg	6g	0g
Generic - Smart Balance Buttery Spread, 1 tbsp	80	0g	9g	0g	0mg	90mg	0g	0g
Pepperidge Farm - Light Style - Soft Wheat - Bread, 2 slice	87	17g	1g	5g	0mg	180mg	2g	3g
Lunch								
Homemade - Unsweetened Iced Tea, 16 oz	0	0g	0g	0g	0mg	5mg	0g	0g
Homemade 1/3 lb Cheeseburger - 1/3 lb Cheeseburger With Lettuce, Tomatoe, Onion, Mayonaise, 1/3 cup	608	39g	39g	34g	104mg	996mg	5g	3g
Dinner								
Cooking Light Recipe - Arugula and Pear Salad With Toasted Walnuts, 1 cups	112	10g	8g	2g	0mg	109mg	0g	0g
Green Giant Fresh - Idaho Potatoes (Medium=148g) Baked Skin and Flesh, 74 g (1 medium)	55	13g	0g	2g	0mg	0mg	1g	1g
Generic - Ice Water W/ Lemon Slices, 16 oz.	10	2g	0g	0g	0mg	0mg	0g	0g
Kirkland Signature - Wild Alaskan Sockeye Salmon (Frozen), 0.5 Portion (170g), 6 oz.	135	0g	7g	16g	48mg	38mg	0g	0g
Smart Balance - Buttery Spread, 1 tbsp	80	0g	9g	0g	0mg	90mg	0g	0g
Snacks								
Generic - Chocolate Birthday Cake, 1 slice	219	29g	9g	5g	0mg	0mg	33g	1g
Generic - Coffee With 30 Ml Skimmed Milk, 1 cup	14	2g	0g	1g	0mg	13mg	1g	0g
TOTAL:	**1,465**	**129g**	**82g**	**69g**	**153mg**	**1,584mg**	**57g**	**8g**

Food Notes

Grilled salmon with dry rub of dill, garlic pepper and kosher salt

EXERCISE	Calories	Minutes	Sets	Reps	Weight
Cardiovascular					
Stair-treadmill ergometer, general	336	31			
TOTALS:	**336**	**31**	**0**	**0**	**0**

Printable Diary for **Mimioriginals**

From: August ▾ 8 ▾ 2011 ▾   Show: ☑ Food Diary   ☑ Food Notes

To: August ▾ 8 ▾ 2011 ▾   ☑ Exercise Diary   ☑ Exercise notes

August 8, 2011

Foods	Calories	Carbs	Fat	Protein	Cholest.	Sodium	Sugars	Fiber
Breakfast								
Generic Fat Free Milk - Non-Fat Milk , 4 oz	45	7g	0g	4g	1mg	63mg	6g	0g
Generic - Smart Balance Buttery Spread, 1 tbsp	80	0g	9g	0g	0mg	90mg	0g	0g
Pepperidge Farm - Light Style - Soft Wheat - Bread, 2 slice	87	17g	1g	5g	0mg	180mg	2g	3g
Coffee - Brewed from grounds, 3 cup (8 fl oz)	7	0g	0g	1g	0mg	14mg	0g	0g
Lunch								
Hummel Bros. - Beef Hot Dog, 1 Hot Dog	150	0g	14g	7g	30mg	480mg	0g	0g
Stop&Shop Light Hot Dog Rolls - Hot Dog Rolls, 1 roll(43g)	80	18g	1g	3g	0mg	180mg	2g	4g
Dinner								
Friendly's - Asian Chicken Salad W/ Sesame Oriental Dressin, 0.5 entree	380	39g	17g	18g	40mg	1,080mg	26g	3g
Friendly Farms - Coffee With Original Creamer, 3 Tbsp	45	6g	3g	0g	0mg	0mg	0g	0g
Snacks								
Friendly's Ice Cream - Maple Walnut, 1 cup	300	32g	18g	6g	50mg	80mg	26g	0g
Starbucks - Unsweetened Iced Brewed Coffee With Nonfat Milk - Venti, 1 serving(s) (24 fl oz ea.)	45	6g	0g	4g	0mg	55mg	6g	0g
Blueberries - Raw, 1 cup	83	21g	0g	1g	0mg	1mg	14g	3g
TOTAL:	**1,302**	**146g**	**63g**	**49g**	**121mg**	**2,223mg**	**82g**	**13g**

Food Notes

Friendly's salad ate half portion, and used half the dressing... added a little at a time ...

Exercise	Calories	Minutes	Sets	Reps	Weight
Cardiovascular					
Stair-treadmill ergometer, general	324	30			
TOTALS:	**324**	**30**	**0**	**0**	**0**

Exercise Notes

1.65 miles

Printable Diary for **Mimioriginals**

From:	August	9	2011	**Show:**	Food Diary	Food Notes	
To:	August	9	2011		Exercise Diary	Exercise notes	

August 9, 2011

FOODS	Calories	Carbs	Fat	Protein	Cholest	Sodium	Sugars	Fiber
Breakfast								
Bisquick Heart Smart - Light and Fluffy Pancakes, 2.25 pancakes	218	0g	3g	0g	30mg	315mg	0g	0g
Oscar Meyer - Center Cut Bacon, 2 slices	47	0g	3g	5g	10mg	180mg	0g	0g
Generic - Smart Balance Buttery Spread, 1 tbsp	80	0g	9g	0g	0mg	90mg	0g	0g
Generic Fat Free Milk - Non-Fat Milk , 4 oz	45	7g	0g	4g	1mg	63mg	6g	0g
Coffee - Brewed from grounds, 3 cup (8 fl oz)	7	0g	0g	1g	0mg	14mg	0g	0g
Lunch								
Hummel Bros. - Beef Hot Dog, 1 Hot Dog	150	0g	14g	7g	30mg	480mg	0g	0g
Stop&Shop Light Hot Dog Rolls - Hot Dog Rolls, 1 roll(43g)	80	18g	1g	3g	0mg	180mg	2g	4g
Generic - Ice Water W/ Lemon Slices, 16 oz.	10	2g	0g	0g	0mg	0mg	0g	0g
Dinner								
Mcdonald's - Asian Chicken Salad W/Crispy Chicken, 3/4 cup	410	45g	20g	28g	45mg	850mg	0g	0g
Mcdonald's - Hot Fudge Sundae, 179 gm	330	54g	10g	8g	25mg	180mg	48g	2g
Mcdonald's - Diet Coke (Medium), 1 serving	0	0g	0g	0g	0mg	30mg	0g	0g
Snacks								
Bryers Ice Cream - Vanilla Fudge Twirl , 1/2 cup	130	17g	6g	2g	15mg	50mg	15g	0g
Eliza-Pitas - Pita Chips, 32 chips	160	0g	0g	0g	0mg	0mg	0g	0g
TOTAL:	1,667	143g	66g	58g	156mg	2,432mg	71g	6g

Food Notes

Big Breakfast Backfired!!! Can't believe the calories in the McDonald's Sundae... next time just the cone!!

EXERCISES	Calories	Minutes	Sets	Reps	Weight
Cardiovascular					
Stair-treadmill ergometer, general	324	30			
TOTALS:	324	30	0	0	0

Exercise Notes

Printable Diary for **Mimioriginals**

From:	August	10	2011	**Show:**	Food Diary	Food Notes
To:	August	10	2011		Exercise Diary	Exercise notes

August 10, 2011

Item	Calories	Carbs	Fat	Protein	Cholest.	Sodium	Sugars	Fiber
Breakfast								
Generic Fat Free Milk - Non-Fat Milk , 4 oz	45	7g	0g	4g	1mg	63mg	6g	0g
Generic - Smart Balance Buttery Spread, 1 tbsp	80	0g	9g	0g	0mg	90mg	0g	0g
Pepperidge Farm - Light Style - Soft Wheat - Bread, 2 slice	87	17g	1g	5g	0mg	180mg	2g	3g
Lunch								
Generic - Canned Red Beets, 1 cup	80	16g	0g	0g	0mg	500mg	12g	2g
Chavrie - Goat's Milk Cheese - Mild, 2 Tbsp	50	1g	4g	3g	20mg	120mg	0g	0g
Nakano - Rice Vinegar (Natural), 1 Tbsp (15 mL)	0	0g	0g	0g	0mg	0mg	0g	0g
Dinner								
Arugula - Raw, 1 cup	5	1g	0g	1g	0mg	5mg	0g	0g
Trader Joe's Organics - Herb Salad Mix, 2 Cups	25	4g	0g	2g	0mg	70mg	0g	2g
Kirkland Signature - Extra Virgin Olive Oil Toscano, 1 tbsp.	120	0g	14g	0g	0mg	0mg	0g	0g
Nakano - Rice Vinegar (Natural), 1 Tbsp (15 mL)	0	0g	0g	0g	0mg	0mg	0g	0g
Tyson Premium 100% All Natural - Boneless/Skinless Chicken Breast, 2.5 ounces	69	0g	0g	14g	34mg	144mg	0g	0g
Ocean Spray Craisins - Crasins 100 Calorie Bags, 1 Tbsp	50	12g	0g	0g	0mg	0mg	9g	1g
Emerald - Glazed Pecans Pecan Pie, 0.13 cup/ 1 oz	75	6g	6g	1g	0mg	55mg	5g	1g
Cucumber - Peeled, raw, 0.5 cup, pared, chopped	8	1g	0g	0g	0mg	1mg	1g	0g
Onions, Raw - Slices - Vegetable, 2 slice, large (38g)	30	8g	0g	0g	0mg	4mg	4g	2g
Snacks								
Kellogg's Special K - Cracker Chips (Backed Snacks) Sea Salt, 60 g (chips)	220	46g	5g	4g	0mg	460mg	2g	6g
Starbucks - Grande Iced Coffee W/ Skim Milk, 16 oz (grande)	110	24g	0g	2g	0mg	30mg	24g	0g
Blueberries - Raw, 1 cup	83	21g	0g	1g	0mg	1mg	14g	3g
TOTAL:	**1,137**	**164g**	**39g**	**37g**	**55mg**	**1,723mg**	**79g**	**20g**

Food Notes

Grilled Chicken Salad - Dry marinate chicken breast in ziplock with dry rosemary, garlic pepper and kosher salt. Place all salad ingredients in salad bowl except for oil and vinegar. Grill chicken and slice in strips. Add oil and vinegar to salad and mix well with hands. Place chicken strips on top and you are ready to enjoy and wonderful salad with protein, great taste and texture!

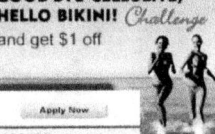

Edit Recipe

Recipe name

Grilled Chicken Salad

Number of servings

Serves 1   people

Ingredients

	Calories	Carbs	Fat	Protein	Sodium	Sugar	
Private Selection - Baby Spring Mix With Herbs Salad, 2 cups (3oz. / 85g)	20	4	0	2	30	2	
Earthbound Farm Organic - Baby Arugula, 3 cups (85g)	30	5	0	3	38	3	
Kirkland Signature - Extra Virgin Olive Oil Toscano, 1 tbsp.	120	0	14	0	0	0	
Nakano - Rice Vinegar (Natural), 1 Tbsp (15 mL)	0	0	0	0	0	0	
Ocean Spray Craisins - Crasins 100 Calorie Bags, 1 Tbsp	60	12	0	0	0	9	
Chavrie - Goat's Milk Cheese - Mild, 2 Tbsp	50	1	4	3	120	0	
Onions - Raw, 0.25 cup, sliced	12	3	0	0	1	1	
Cucumber - Peeled, raw, 0.5 cup, pared, chopped	8	1	0	0	1	1	
Emerald - Glazed Pecans Pecan Pie, 0.13 cup/ 1 oz	75	6	6	1	55	5	
Tyson Premium 100% All Natural - Boneless/Skinless Chicken Breast, 2.5 ounces	69	0	0	14	144	0	
Spices - Rosemary, dried, 1 tbsp	11	2	1	0	2	0	

Add Ingredient

Total:	445	34	25	23	391	21
Per Serving:	445	34	25	23	391	21

Would you like to submit this recipe to the MyFitnessPal recipe database?
No   Yes

SAVE CHANGES   CANCEL

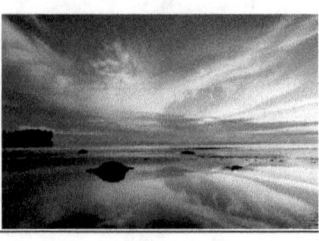

Carol Ann's 1300 a day calories
All calories are approximate
Breakfast

1 egg w/ spinach –(70 calories)
1 slice/ 3 oz. of cinnamon bun- (306. 1 calories)
¼ c. fresh pineapple sliced- (12.5 calories)
1 c. of black tea
total: 376 calories

Lunch
1 Yoplait (110 calories)
1 Macoun's apple-80 cal.
1 oz of Vt. Cheddar cheese-110 cal.
1 c. black tea
Total: 300 calories

dinner
½ egg roll (150 calories)
2 steamed dumplings (50 calories)
1 c. chinese chicken & broccoli-(280 calories)
½ c. brown rice-1/2 c. – (112 calories)
total dinner 592 calories

snack
½ cup of fresh sliced pineapple + 1 tsp of non-fat plain yogurt (35 calories)

approximately 1306 calories on Monday
//
Tuesday breakfast
1/2 c. of Cherrios-50 cal
½ c. skim milk -45 cal
3 tbs. dried cranberries-110 cal

¼ c. fresh frozen blueberries-41 cal
½ grapefruit peeled and seeded- 41 cal.
Approx. 307 calories

Lunch
1 slice of wheat bread (100)
1.9 oz of ptly. skimmed Jarelsburg cheese (200)
2 slices of tomato
salt & pepper & dill weed
4 baby carrots (35 cal.)
1 diet coke
approx. 335

Dinner
1 ¼ c. of pasta (250 cal.)
2 c. of H.M. meat (93/7) & maranara sauce (approx. 222 cal.)
2 c. of salad with 2 tbs. of Balsamic Vinegar -60 calories
approx. 530 cal.

snack
½ c. fresh cut pineapple
Tot. calories : 1199
//
Breakfast:
1 c. Oat squares –120 calories
½ banana   -85 calories
1 c. skim milk -90 calories
black tea
total   295 cal.

Lunch
Yogurt- 110 calories
1 Macoun -80 cal.
Total 190 calories

Dinner
4 oz. baked in lemon haddock—150 cal.
2 small red potatoes-220 cal.
½ c. of corn—72 cal.
½ c. spinach in 1 tsp. oil & garlic -25 calories

2 4 oz glasses of chardonnay—160 calories
2-c. of salad (romaine, cukes, tomato, spinach w/balsamic vinegar only)
total calories 502 calories

grand tot calories –1831 calories

Breakfast
2 slices French wheat toast
1 egg white
1 whole canned peach
tea w/ lemon
total

Lunch
Yoplait light
LWWE chips
1 HM gluten & wheat free cranberry nut scone
total

Dinner
1 ½ c. pasta
1 c. broccoli & cauliflowerts & garnish of tomato & cilantro
1 tbs. of pesto
2-4 oz glass of Merlot
Total
Grand Total

Breakfast
2 flat rye rounds, Egg white, a slice of cheese, and chopped veggies (a

black coffee
Total
Lunch
6 ritiz crackers
2 oz of Jarslberg lite swiss cheese
1 Macoun apple
1 c. of black tea w/ lemon.
Total

Dinner
1 ¼ c. of pasta   (250 cal.)
2 c. of H.M. meat (93/7) & maranara sauce   222 cal.)
2 c. of salad with 2 tbs. of Balsamic Vinegar   -60 calories
                                                   approx. 530 cal.

Snack
1 c. fresh pineapple   78 calories

Grand total   1274 calories

1404 Calorie Meal Plan

Breakfast

2 slices light bread, toasted	80 cal
1 Tbsp peanut butter, spread thinly on toast	95 cal
1 medium banana, sliced (on top of peanut butter)	85 cal
black coffee	0 cal

Morning snack

3 Crisp 'n Light 7 Grain Wasa flatbread/crackers	60 cal
½ cup nonfat cottage cheese	80 cal
large mug hot tea sweetened with 2 tsp Splenda	4 cal

Lunch

1 frozen meal, like Lean Cuisine, etc. (choose lower salt, limit calories)	300 cal
4 spears steamed broccoli, sprinkled with lemon juice	50 cal
20 seedless grapes	70 cal
tea, water or coffee	0 cal

Afternoon snack

(1) 100-calorie serving of popcorn	100 cal
tea, water or coffee	0 cal

Dinner

2 slices light rye bread	100 cal
2 oz extra lean 5% fat ham	70 cal
2 slices roasted peppers packed in water	20 cal
1 tsp mustard	5 cal
1 cup shredded cabbage with 2 Tbsp light Italian dressing	85 cal
2 cups watermelon, peeled and cubed	100 cal
water with lemon	0 cal

Dessert

1 Nonni's chocolate "Decadence" biscotti	100 cal
tea or coffee	0 cal

1442 Calorie Meal Plan

Breakfast
French toast:
   ▲ 2 slices light bread, 1 egg beaten with cinnamon/Splenda/vanilla   155 cal
   ▲ Brown on hot griddle prepared with cooking spray
2 Tbsp sugar free maple syrup   50 cal
10 seedless grapes   35 cal
black coffee   0 cal

Morning snack
1 cup light fruit cocktail   120 cal
large mug hot tea sweetened with 2 tsp Splenda   4 cal

Lunch
1 cup butternut squash soup   90 cal
10 seasoned croutons   50 cal
1 medium apple, sliced   100 cal
1 light Babybel cheese round   50 cal
tea, water or coffee   0 cal

Afternoon snack
2 Tbsp hummus   50 cal
6 baby carrots   25 cal
tea, water or coffee   0 cal

Dinner
4 oz lean sirloin steak, grilled   200 cal
oven fries:
   ▲ 1 small potato cut into wedges   135 cal
   ▲ coat with cooking spray and roast in hot oven
2 Tbsp ketchup   40 cal
½ cup each, sliced: onion, mushrooms and zucchini   40 cal
   ▲ saute with 1 tsp olive oil, salt, pepper   40 cal

Dessert
½ cup Edy's light vanilla ice cream   100 cal

1458 Calorie Meal Plan

Breakfast

1 serving cooked hot cereal made with nonfat milk and 2 tsp Splenda	214 cal
1 medium banana	100 cal
black coffee	0 cal

Mid-morning snack

1 "thin" bagel, toasted	110 cal
1 light Babybel cheese round, sliced, placed on the bagel	50 cal
large mug hot tea sweetened with 2 tsp Splenda	4 cal

Lunch

1 light English muffin, toasted	100 cal
1 large egg, poached in microwave (placed on the muffin)	75 cal
1 round slice Canadian bacon, warmed (on top of the egg)	40 cal
1 slice 2% milk Kraft single cheese (on top of the bacon)	50 cal
20 seedless grapes	70 cal
tea, water or coffee	0 cal

Mid-afternoon snack

1 large orange	85 cal
tea, water or coffee	0 cal

Dinner

4 oz boneless skinless chicken, grilled with lemon juice, salt, pepper	200 cal
4 cups lettuce, onion, red bell pepper, grape tomatoes (combined)	100 cal
4 Tbsp FF ranch	80 cal
steamed asparagus	40 cal
water with lemon	0 cal

Dessert

4 saltine crackers (unsalted)	50 cal
1 Tbsp strawberry Simply fruit, divided	40 cal
1 cup hot cocoa, light-no sugar added	50 cal

1392 Calorie Meal Plan

Breakfast
1 poached egg	75 cal
1 light English muffin	100 cal
1 cup watermelon, peeled and cubed	50 cal
black coffee	0 cal

Morning snack
3 Crisp 'n Light 7 Grain Wasa flatbread/crackers	60 cal
1 light Laughing Cow cheese wedge	35 cal
large mug hot tea sweetened with 2 tsp Splenda	4 cal

Lunch
4 cups salad (mixed lettuce, onion, peppers, etc.)	100 cal
½ of 6 oz. can tuna packed in water, drained	88 cal
1 large tomato, cut into wedges	30 cal
4 Tbsp fat free Thousand Island dressing	80 cal
1 slice light bread toasted, cut into 8 wedges	40 cal
tea, water or coffee	0 cal

Afternoon snack
1 medium banana	100 cal
tea, water or coffee	0 cal

Dinner
4 oz baked sole (with 1 tsp olive oil, salt, pepper)	175 cal
1 cup cooked carrots (with 1 tsp light butter)	85 cal
1 cup cooked spinach (with 1 tsp olive oil, salt, pepper)	80 cal
1 medium baked potato (with 1 tsp light butter, salt, pepper)	175 cal
water with lemon	0 cal

Dessert
½ cup sugar-free fat free pudding	70 cal
1 square graham cracker (broken up added to pudding)	30 cal
2 Tbsp Cool Whip Free	15 cal
tea or coffee	0 cal

1310 Calorie Meal Plan

Breakfast
1 ¼ cup Rice Krispies with 2 tsp Splenda   134 cal
1 cup nonfat milk   90 cal
1 large orange   85 cal
black coffee   0 cal

Morning snack
1 serving light fat free yogurt   100 cal
1/8 cup Fiber One cereal (mixed into yogurt)   15 cal
large mug hot tea sweetened with 2 tsp Splenda   4 cal

Lunch
1 cup Progresso Light Vegetable Noodle soup   60 cal
½ "thin" bagel   55 cal
1 slice light Swiss cheese   70 cal
20 seedless grapes   70 cal
tea, water or coffee   0 cal

Afternoon snack
(1) 100 cal snack-bag (chocolate chip) cookies   100 cal
tea, water or coffee   0 cal

Dinner
1 cup whole wheat pasta, cooked   175 cal
½ cup marinara sauce   80 cal
1 cup chopped broccoli, steamed (mix into pasta and sauce)   50 cal
1 Tbsp grated Parmesan cheese   22 cal
2 cups lettuce, onion, red bell pepper, grape tomatoes (combined)   50 cal
2 Tbsp fat free Red Wine Vinaigrette (Wishbone)   35 cal
water with lemon   0 cal

Dessert
1 baked apple (with cinnamon and Splenda)   100 cal

2 Tbsp Cool Whip Free   15 cal

CHAPTER SEVEN

RECIPES

In loving memory of Carol Elizabeth Meier

CARMELA'S CROCK-POT
MEATBALLS AND TOMATO SAUCE

Meatballs

1 lb. ground (93%) turkey .... 600 cal.

4 slices lite (50 cal) bread .... 200 cal.

1 egg .... 75 cal.

2 Tbsp grated Romano cheese .... 40 cal.

Garlic powder, basil, salt, black pepper

Total cal. = 815 raw, Total weight = 21 ozs. raw, Makes 16 (1.3 ozs. raw) meatballs @ 51 cal. each

Tomato Sauce

2 large cans crushed tomatoes (28 ozs. each @260 cal.) .... .520 cal.

2 cans tomato paste (6 ozs. each @150 cal.) .... .300 cal.

Garlic powder, basil, salt, black pepper .... negligible

Total cal. = 820 cal., Total volume = 9.5 cups, 1 cup = 86 cal.

Directions

1. Moisten bread with water and break into small pieces. Place in large bowl with other meatball ingredients. Gently mix together with hands until blended (do not overwork it).

2. Using wet hands, divide meatball mixture into 16 equal amounts (using scale is best). Form into meatballs and place on cookie sheet sprayed with cooking oil. Add 1 spray of cooking oil on the top of each raw meatball.

3. Bake in 375 degree oven for 20 minutes, flip meatballs over, then bake another 5-10 minutes until brown.

4. Mix tomato paste and crushed tomatoes in slow cooker pot. Blend in seasonings.

5. Add cooked meatballs to tomato mixture.

6. Cook on low 6-8 hours.

7. Serve with pasta (count extra calories)

Helpful Hints

- 1 cup = 16 Tbsp   6 ozs. paste = 10 Tbsp = 1.25 cups, x 2 cans = 2.5 cups
- 28 ozs. tomatoes = 3.5 cups, x 2 cans = 7 cups
- Use a whisk to thoroughly mix tomatoes and paste together
- Line cookie sheet with parchment paper for easier cleanup.

CAROL ELIZABETH'S ASPARAGUS PASTA
8 servings

Ingredients

2 lbs. asparagus, sliced diagonally into 1" pieces .... 192 cal. @ 6 cal. per oz.

¼ cup (12 tsp.) Dijon mustard .... 60 cal. @ 5 cal. per tsp.

¼ cup olive oil .... 482 cal. @ 1930 cal. per cup

½ cup thinly sliced shallots .... approx 25 cal.

2 cloves garlic, minced .... 8 cal.

1 tsp. anchovy paste .... 10 cal. @ 30 cal. per Tbsp

½ tsp. thyme .... negligible

¼ cup chopped parsley .... 5 cal.

1 lb. very thin spaghetti or pasta of your choice .... 1685 cal.

Salt and pepper to taste .... negligible

Total approximately 2467 cal. or 308 cal. per serving.

Directions

1. In large pot of boiling water, cook asparagus until tender (about 3 minutes).
2. Combine mustard, olive oil, shallots, garlic, anchovy paste, thyme and parsley. Set dressing aside.
3. Cook pasta according to package directions. Drain but reserve 1 cup of the cooking water.
4. Combine pasta with dressing mix and asparagus. Mix well, adding some pasta water if it is too dry.
5. Season with salt and pepper.

CARMELA'S CHICKEN PARMIGIANO MADE EASY

4 servings @ 303 cal per serving

Ingredients

1/3 cup breadcrumbs	128 cal. @ 385 ca.l per cup
4 Tbsp grated Parmesan cheese	88 cal. @ 22 cal per Tbsp
½ tsp. dried basil	negligible
¼ tsp. garlic powder	negligible
1/8 tsp. black pepper	negligible
Dash salt	negligible
1 large egg	75 cal.
4 skinless boneless chicken breasts (about 4 ozs. each)	400 cal.
1 Tbsp olive oil	120 cal.
1 cup jarred marinara sauce	185 cal.
3 ozs. shredded part-skim mozzarella	216 cal. @ 72 cal. per oz.

Directions

1. Mix breadcrumbs, cheese, basil, garlic powder, black pepper and salt in a plastic bag.
2. Beat egg in a bowl until frothy.
3. Pound each chicken breast to about ½ inch thick.
4. Dip each breast into the egg and then shake in the plastic bag to coat with the seasoned breadcrumbs.
5. Heat the oil in a large nonstick skillet over medium heat.
6. Add the chicken to the skillet and cook about 5 minutes per side until browned and cooked through.
7. Spoon the marinara sauce evenly over each chicken breast. Sprinkle the shredded mozzarella over the sauce.
8. Cover the pan and continue to cook over low heat for another 5 minutes to melt the cheese.

Note

- To make it a one-pot" meal, add canned or frozen (cooked) string beans and/or mushrooms to the pan when you add the marinara. Let it heat through all together (count extra calories).
- Serve with pasta or rice on the side (count extra calories).

CAROL ELIZABETH'S CHICKEN SMOTHERED IN VEGETABLES

4 servings

Ingredients

4 boneless skinless chicken breast halves (4 ozs. each) ..... 520 cal. @ 130 cal. per 4 ozs.

¼ cup unbleached white flour .... 114 cal. @ 455 cal. per cup

½ tsp. salt .... negligible

1/8 tsp. ground pepper .... negligible

1/8 cup olive oil .... 240 cal. @ 240 cal. per 1 oz.

1 clove garlic, minced .... 4 cal.

¾ cup sliced onion .... 36 cal.

½ green pepper, sliced .... approx. 20 cal.

1 cup sliced mushrooms .... 15 cal.

1 tsp. oregano .... negligible

8 cherry tomatoes .... 24 cal.

Total approximately 973 cal. or 243 cal. per serving.

Directions

1. Preheat oven to 375 degrees.

2. Spray shallow baking pan with cooking spray or grease with margarine.

3. Cut each chicken breast into 4 pieces.

4. Mix flour, salt and pepper in plastic bag. Coat chicken with flour mixture by shaking in bag.

5. Place coated chicken in baking pan and grind additional black pepper over it.

6. In large skillet saute garlic and onion in olive oil until soft.

7. Stir in green pepper, mushrooms and oregano. Cook for 1 minute.

8. Add tomatoes to skillet and stir to mix.

9. Pour vegetables over chicken and bake 40 minutes until cooked.

CAROL ELIZABETH'S CREAMY FETTUCCINE WITH VEGETABLES

6 servings

Ingredients

1 cup sliced carrots . . . . 50 cal.

1 cup sliced zucchini . . . . 18 cal.

1 cup broccoli florets . . . . 30 cal.

1 cup string beans (cut in half) . . . . 34 cal.

8 ozs. fettuccine . . . . 840 cal. @ 105 cal per oz.

1 ½ cups low fat cottage cheese . . . . 240 cal. @ 160 cal. per cup

2/3 cup skim milk . . . . 60 cal. @ 90 cal. per cup

2 tsp. Basil . . . . negligible

¼ cup chopped parsley . . . . 5 cal.

Total approximately 1277 cal. or 213 cal. per serving.

Directions

1. Steam carrots, zucchini, broccoli and green beans until tender. Put in serving bowl.
2. Cook pasta according to package directions. Drain and set aside to cool.
3. Using a blender or food processor, puree cottage cheese until smooth. Blend in skim milk, basil and parsley.
4. Combine vegetables and pasta.
5. Pour sauce over pasta and vegetables. Mix until well-covered.
6. Serve at room temperature.

CAROL'S MEATBALLS FOR A CROWD
Serves about 15
Approx. 65 cal. per meatball

Ingredients

1 ½ lbs. of 90/93% lean ground beef (@ 51 cal. per cooked oz.)

½ to ¾ of a cup of oat bran (@ 120 cal. per ¼ cup for Hodgson's Mill Brand)

½ or ¼ cup chopped green pepper

½ cup or ¼ cup finely chopped onion

1 large clove freshly minced garlic

1 tsp. oregano

1 Tbsp chopped parsley

Salt and pepper to taste

Directions

1. Mix all ingredients together with your clean hands or gloved hands for 5 minutes. If you feel it's too dry add 1 tbs. of water for easy handling.
2. Keep mixing it until you can roll them into balls. Roll to desired size.
3. Place meatballs into Pam-sprayed shallow baking dish or cookie sheet.
4. Line the dish with foil for easy clean-up.
5. Bake at 350 degrees until brown (about 20 minutes depending on thickness).
6. When done, drain on paper towel if needed, and place into your favorite sauce (count extra calories).
7. Cook together with sauce about 30 minutes or until flavors have married.

JENNIE'S CHICKEN
4 servings
Approx. 290 cal. per serving (if made with wine)

Ingredients

1 pkg. skinless chicken breasts, halved (with/without bone) … 184 cal. per 4 ozs. baked

1 medium-large onion sliced and diced . . . . 56 cal.

2 cloves of minced garlic . . . . 8 cal.

1 green pepper, chopped . . . . 30 cal.

1 lb of sliced mushrooms (Baby Bellas) . . . . 10 cal. per ½ cup

1 tbsp of oregano . . . . negligible

1 tsp of rosemary . . . . negligible

2 cans (14.5 ozs. each) diced tomatoes . . . . 25 cal. per can

Salt and pepper to taste . . . . negligible

Optional: ¼ cup (2 ozs.) red wine . . . . 85 cal.

Optional: wine vinegar . . . . 0 cal.

Directions

1. Line a 9"x13" cake pan with foil.

2. Place halved chicken breasts on foiled pan.

3. Put all the rest of the ingredients on top of the mixture.

4. Cover tightly with foil.

5. Bake at 350 degrees for at least 1 hour.

6. Serve with a green veggie over brown rice or noodles (count extra calories).

7. Spoon juice over veggies and rice.

CARMELA'S VEGETABLE CHILI

After trying several different recipes, this is my version...you can eat it right away or make it a day ahead...it gets better as all the flavors blend.
Total 1598 cal. • 10 servings @ 160 cal. • 12 servings @ 133 cal.

Ingredients

2 Tbsp olive oil . . . . 240 cal.

1 cup carrots, sliced very thin . . . . 50 cal .

2 large stalks celery, sliced into ½ inch pieces . . . . 18 cal.

1 medium onion, chopped . . . . 46 cal.

1 large green bell pepper, seeded and chopped . . . . 33 cal.

1 large red bell pepper, seeded and chopped . . . . 43 cal.

2 cloves garlic, minced . . . . 8 cal.

1 envelope hot chili mix (1.25 ozs.) . . . . 120 cal.

1 (28 ozs.) can diced tomatoes, with juice (do not drain) . . . . 140 cal.

2 cups corn (canned, drained) . . . . 260 cal.

6 cups assorted canned beans, drained and rinsed* . . . . 630 cal.

2 tsp. Worcestershire sauce . . . . 10 cal.

Use whatever beans you like – try a mix of white, pink, pintos, small red kidneys, etc.

Directions

1. Heat oil in large pan and saute carrots, celery, onions, peppers and garlic until soft.

2. Mix in chili seasoning, tomatoes, corn and beans.

3. Simmer all together about 45-60 minutes, until heated through and flavors have all blended.

4. Add extra chili seasoning if you like it extra spicy.

Note

Optional additions (count extra calories)

• Toppings (sour cream, shredded cheddar, etc.)

• Rice, cooked

CAROL ELIZABETH'S
LEMON MUSTARD CHICKEN

6 servings

Ingredients

6 skinless chicken breast halves (4 ozs. each) ....780 cal. @ 130 cal. per 4 os.z

¼ cup margarine (2 oz) ....400 ca.l @ 200 cal. per oz.

3 Tbsp dijon mustard ....45 cal. @ 5 cal. per tsp.

3 Tbsp lemon juice ....approx 10 cal.

1 tsp. tarragon ....negligible

½ tsp. salt ....negligible

Total approximately 1235 cal. or 205 cal. per serving.

Directions

1. Preheat oven to 375 degrees.
2. Place chicken in shallow baking pan.
3. Met margarine in small saucepan. Stir in mustard, lemon juice, tarragon and salt. Pour over chicken.
4. Bake chicken for 45 minutes or until cooked.
5. Spoon sauce over chicken and serve.

CAROL ELIZABETH'S PEPPERY CHICKEN
Roasted or Grilled
8 servings

Ingredients

8 skinless chicken breast halves (4 ozs. each) ...... 1040 cal. @ 130 cal. per 4 ozs.

2 Tbsp olive oil .... 240 cal. @ 120 cal. per Tbsp

2 Tbsp soy sauce .... 20 cal. @ 10 cal. per Tbsp

2 Tbsp honey .... 130 cal. @ 65 cal. per Tbsp

½ tsp. thyme .... negligible

½ tsp. paprika .... negligible

¼ tsp. cayenne pepper .... negligible

1 Tbsp white vinegar .... negligible

½ tsp. allspice .... negligible

1 tsp. ground black pepper .... negligible

2 cups sliced mushrooms .... 30 cal.

Total approximately 1460 cal. or 183 cal. per serving.

Directions

1. Place chicken in shallow casserole.
2. Combine oil, soy sauce, honey, thyme, paprika, cayenne pepper, vinegar, allspice and black pepper and pour over chicken.
3. Marinate 1 hour.

Baking

- Preheat oven to 375 degrees.
- Bake chicken until almost cooked (30-45 minutes).
- Surround chicken with sliced mushrooms. Spoon chicken juices/sauce over them.
- Bake another 5-10 minutes until mushrooms are done.

Grilling

- Remove breasts from marinade and grill until cooked.
- Add mushrooms to marinade and simmer approximately 5 to10 minutes until cooked.
- Use marinade to baste chicken as well.

ELIZABETH'S MEATLOAF
1217 total cal.
8 servings @ 152 cal. per serving

Ingredients

1 small onion, finely chopped .... 30 cal.

1 small carrot, grated .... 20 cal.

½ cup celery, finely chopped .... 7 cal.

Salt, pepper, garlic powder to taste .... negligible

1 ¼ lbs. 93% lean ground beef .... 800 cal. @ 40 cal. per oz.

3 slices light white bread .... 120 cal. @ 40 cal. per slice

1 large egg .... 75 cal.

3 Tbsp Worcestershire sauce .... 30 cal .

1 can (14 ozs.) bean sprouts, drained .... 45 cal.

6 Tbsp ketchup, divided .... 0 cal. @15 cal. per Tbsp

Directions

1. Preheat oven to 350 degrees.
2. Coat nonstick frying pan with cooking spray.
3. Add onion, carrot and celery to skillet. Season generously with salt, pepper and garlic powder.
4. Saute vegetables over medium heat until softened, about 5-6 minutes. Set aside to cool.
5. Moisten bread with water and tear into little pieces. Set aside.
6. In large bowl, mix together beef, moistened bread, cooled vegetables, bean sprouts, egg, 3 Tbsp of the ketchup and Worcestershire sauce.
7. Shape into loaf and place into baking pan which was prepared with nonstick cooking spray.
8. Spread top of meat loaf with remaining 3 Tbsp ketchup.
9. Bake uncovered for about 60 minutes or until done.

Note

- Bean sprouts are bland so be sure to generously season the vegetables and/or the meat mixture before you bake it.
- Bean sprouts bring added moisture; recommend baking in shallow baking pan or dish, uncovered.

CAROL ELIZABETH'S
APRICOT CHICKEN DIVINE

8 servings

Ingredients

2 Tbsp margarine .... 200 cal. @ 100 cal. per Tbsp

2 Tbsp olive oil .... 240 cal. @ 120 cal. per Tbsp

8 skinless chicken breast halves (4 ozs. each) .... 1040 cal. @ 130 cal. per 4 oz

½ cup unbleached white flour .... 228 cal. @ 455 cal. per cup

1 tsp. salt .... negligible

½ cup (8 Tbsp) apricot preserves .... 400 cal. @ 50 cal. per Tbsp

1 Tbsp Dijon mustard .... 15 cal. @ 5 cal. per tsp

½ cup nonfat yogurt .... 63 cal. @ 125 cal. per cup

Optional: 2 Tbsp slivered almonds

Total approximately 2186 cal. or 273 cal. per serving.

Directions

1. Preheat oven to 375 degrees.
2. Melt margarine with olive oil in shallow baking pan.
3. Mix flour and salt in plastic bag. Shake chicken in bag to coat with flour.
4. Place chicken in baking pan in single layer. Bake 25 minutes.
5. Combine apricot preserves, mustard and yogurt.
6. Spread apricot mixture over chicken and bake an additional 30 minutes until cooked.

Optional: Sprinkle with slivered almonds before serving (count extra calories).

CARMELA'S SHRIMP WITH VEGETABLES
4 servings @ 236 cal. per serving

Ingredients

1 Tbsp olive oil .... 120 cal.

2 cloves garlic, minced .... 8 cal.

1 medium onion cut into 1-inch pieces .... 46 cal.

1 large green bell pepper cut into 1-inch pieces .... 33 cal.

1 can diced tomatoes with juice (14 ozs.) .... 70 cal.

6 ozs. tomato paste .... 156 cal.

1 cup water .... 0 cal.

1 small can mushrooms, drained .... 33 cal.

½ tsp. basil .... negligible

Salt and black pepper to taste .... negligible

⅛ tsp. cayenne pepper (optional) .... negligible

1 lb. raw shrimp .... 480 cal.

Cook garlic and onion in olive oil about 1 minute over medium heat.

Directions

1. Add green pepper and cook another 3 -5 minutes until tender.
2. Add diced tomatoes, tomato paste, water, mushrooms, basil, salt, black pepper and cayenne (optional).
3. Mix well and simmer over low heat about 10 minutes.
4. Add shrimp to simmering sauce and cook until shrimp are opaque and just cooked through (about 5-6 minutes).
5. Serve with pasta or rice (count additional calories).

CARMELA'S TOMATO AND BASIL FRITTATA
4 servings

Ingredients

8 large eggs . . . . 600 cal. @ 75 cal. per egg

1 cup grape tomatoes, cut in half . . . . approx 30 cal.

¼ cup fresh basil, chopped or torn into pieces . . . . 2 cal. @ 1 cal. per 5 leaves

4 Tbsp (2 ozs.) grated Romano cheese . . . . 220 cal. @ 100 cal. per oz.

Salt and pepper to taste . . . . negligible

Total approximately 852 cal. or 213 cal. per serving.

Directions

1. Beat eggs in bowl. Stir in cheese, basil salt and pepper. Fold in tomatoes.

2. Coat nonstick skillet with cooking spray and place over medium heat.

3. Pour in egg mixture and cook for about a minute until the eggs start to set on the bottom.

4. Use a spatula to lift edges of the frittata so the uncooked egg runs underneath into the bottom of the hot pan. Continue to cook this way for about another minute until the top of the frittata is wet but not runny.

5. Lower the heat and cover the pan. Cook about 5 more minutes until top is set.

6. Alternatively, to finish the frittata, you can set it in a preheated 350 degree oven, uncovered, until the top is set (about 5 minutes) as long as your skillet is oven proof.

LYNN'S PASTA E FAGIOLI CON CARNE
8 servings (164 cal./serving)
6 servings (219 cal./serving)

Ingredients

2 cups drained and rinsed cannellini beans .... 420 cal. @ 105 cal./half cup

½ lb. sweet Italian turkey sausage .... 352 cal. @ 44 cal./oz.

1 medium onion, cut into ½ inch dice .... 46 cal.

1 medium stalk celery with leaves, thinly sliced .... 6 cal.

2 medium carrots, peeled and thinly sliced .... 50 cal.

2 large cloves garlic, minced .... 8 cal.

1 tsp. finely chopped rosemary (or ½ tsp. dried crushed) .... negligible

1 can (28 ozs.) Italian plum tomatoes with juice (crushed) .... 140 cal.

Salt and pepper to taste .... negligible

¾ cup small pasta (elbows or ditalini) .... 262 cal. @ 350 cal./cup

2 cups beef broth .... 0 cal. @ 15 cal./cup

Optional: 1 Tbsp Parmigiano Reggiano cheese per serving .. add 22 cal. per Tbsp

Directions

1. Heat oil in large soup pot over medium heat. Add onion, celery, carrot, garlic, rosemary and sausage (out of the casing). Saute uncovered until sausage begins to brown, about 10 minutes. Reduce heat to low and add tomatoes, salt and pepper. Cook until the liquid evaporates (about 15 minutes).

2. Prepare pasta according to package directions.

3. Add the beans and broth to the soup pot. Raise the heat, bring to a boil, then reduce the heat to a simmer. Cover and cook another 15 minutes. If more broth is needed, add a little more but remember this is supposed to be a thick soup. Drain the pasta and add to the soup, stir well.

4. If served with grated cheese add extra calories as noted above.

Note

Soup can be frozen before the pasta is added. Add the pasta when you defrost and re-heat the soup later.

CAROL ELIZABETH'S TUNA PASTA BAKE

4 servings

Ingredients

2 tsp. vegetable oil .... 90 cal.

½ cup chopped onion .... 35 cal.

1 garlic clove, minced .... 4 cal.

1 can (8 ozs.) tomato sauce .... 80 cal.

½ tsp. oregano .... negligible

2 cups cooked spaghetti .... 450 cal.

1 can tuna (7 ozs. in water), drained and flaked .... 220 cal.

½ cup cooked peas .... 60 cal.

1 cup low fat cottage cheese .... 160 cal.

1 egg slightly beaten .... 75 cal.

¼ tsp. pepper .... negligible

1 ½ tsp. wheat germ .... 13 cal. @ 25 cal. per Tbsp

Total approximately 1187 cal. or 297 cal. per serving.

Directions

1. Preheat oven to 375 degrees. Coat 1 ½ quart baking dish with cooking spray.

2. Heat oil in small saucepan over medium-high heat.

3. Add onion and garlic. Cook about 3 minutes stirring occasionally.

4. Add tomato sauce and oregano. Cook together about 15 minutes. Set aside.

5. Cook spaghetti according to package directions, but do not add salt.

6. Drain spaghetti and place in medium bowl. Add tuna and peas. Mix well.

7. In another small bowl combine cottage cheese, egg and pepper.

8. Pour cheese mixture over spaghetti in bowl and mix well.

9. Place spaghetti-cheese mixture in prepared baking dish.

10. Pour prepared tomato sauce over the top and sprinkle with wheat germ.

11. Bake about 30 minutes.

CAROL ELIZABETH'S MEXICAN TORTILLA CASSEROLE

6 servings

Ingredients

1 Tbsp canola oil	120 cal.
1 cup chopped onion	70 cal.
½ chopped green pepper	20 cal.
1 garlic clove, minced	4 cal.
1 can (14.5 ozs.) stewed tomatoes	100 cal.
¼ cup dry red wine	50 cal.
1 tsp. chili powder	negligible
¼ tsp. ground cumin	negligible
¼ tsp. ground black pepper	negligible
6 corn tortillas	420 cal. @ 70 cal. each
1 cup part skim ricotta	340 cal.
1 large egg white	17 cal.
1 ¼ cup kidney beans, rinsed and drained	263 cal. @ 210 cal. per cup
¼ cup part skim mozzarella, grated	80 cal.
1 Tbsp Parmesan cheese	20 cal.

Total approximately 1504 cal. or 251 cal. per serving.

Directions

1. Heat oil in medium saucepan over medium-high heat.
2. Add onion, green pepper and garlic. Cook about 3 minutes.
3. Add tomatoes, wine, chili powder, cumin and black pepper. Bring to a boil, reduce heat, cover and simmer for about 20 minutes, stirring occasionally.
4. Preheat oven to 350 degrees.
5. In small bowl blend ricotta and egg white until smooth.
6. Coat bottom of 2 quart casserole with nonstick cooking spray.
7. Spread a small amount of prepared tomato sauce in bottom of casserole.
8. Lay 3 tortillas over sauce to cover.
9. Spread half the ricotta mixture over the tortillas.
10. Spread half the beans over the ricotta mixture.
11. Spread half the remaining sauce over the beans.
12. Repeat layers to complete the casserole.
13. Top with mozzarella and Parmesan cheeses.
14. Bake 30-40 minutes until done.

GRANDMA'S GREEN BEANS
8 servings (133 cal./serving)
6 servings (177 cal. /serving)

Ingredients

1 lb. green beans, washed and cut .... 144 cal. @ 9 cal./oz.

2 medium potatoes, peeled and cubed .... 328 cal. @ 164 each

2 cups of your favorite tomato sauce .... 320 cal. @ 80 cal. per half cup

1 small onion, finely diced .... 30 cal.

1 clove garlic, minced (optional) .... 4 cal.

2 Tbsp olive oil .... 238 cal. @ 119 per Tbsp

Salt and pepper to taste .... negligible

1 cup water .... 0 cal.

Directions

1. In saucepan saute onions and garlic (optional) in olive oil at medium heat.

2. When onions are translucent, add in green beans and mix to coat.

3. Cover mixture in the saucepan with your choice of sauce and add diced potatoes.

4. Mix all ingredients together.

CARMELA'S ITALIAN WEDDING SOUP
10 servings @ 137 cal.

Meatball Ingredients

¾ lb. 93 % lean ground turkey .... 480 cal.

2 slices light white bread cut into small pieces .... 80 cal.

1 tsp. garlic powder .... negligible

1 Tbsp dried basil .... negligible

4 Tbsp grated Parmesan cheese .... 88 cal.

2 extra-large egg whites .... 32 cal.

1 tsp. salt .... negligible

½ tsp. black pepper .... negligible

Soup Ingredients

2 Tbsp olive oil .... 240 cal.

1 small yellow onion, minced .... 30 cal.

2 large carrots, cut into ¼ inch pieces .... 60 cal.

2 large stalks celery, cut into ¼ inch pieces .... 20 cal.

10 cups light reduced sodium fat-free chicken broth .... 50 cal.

2 ozs. small pasta like acini di pepe .... 210 cal.

1 small head escarole, washed, trimmed, steamed and drained .... 80 cal.

Optional: 1 Tbsp grated parmesan cheese per serving .... count extra 22 cal.

1. Preheat the oven to 350 degrees.

2. Meatballs: mix together the ground turkey, bread, garlic powder, basil, grated cheese, egg whites, salt, and pepper. Roll into 1 inch meatballs and place on a sheet pan lined with parchment paper. Bake for about 30 minutes, until cooked through and lightly browned. Set aside.

3. Soup: heat the olive oil over medium-low heat in a large soup pot. Add the onion, carrots, and celery. Saute until softened, approx 10 minutes. Add the chicken broth and bring to a boil.

4. Add the cooked meatballs and the pasta to the broth and cook for 6 to 8 minutes, until the pasta is tender. Stir in the previously steamed escarole. Reduce heat and simmer all together for 10 minutes.

5. Ladle into soup bowls and sprinkle each serving with 1 Tbsp grated Parmesan cheese (optional).

6. Cover pan and simmer at medium heat until vegetables are tender (about 45 minutes). Stir frequently.

7. About halfway through cook-time, add in 1 cup of water.

CARMELA'S BREAKFAST IN A MUG

Here's a quick and easy recipe for breakfast...or for any meal!

Ingredients

2 large eggs, beaten ....150 cal.

1 wedge Laughing Cow Light (any flavor) ....35 cal.

2 Tbsp Hormel (real) bacon bits ....50 cal.

Salt and pepper to taste

Directions

1. Coat microwave-safe mug with cooking spray.

2. Add all ingredients to mug and stir to combine.

3. Microwave uncovered on high for 1 minute; stir.

4. Continue to microwave for 1 to 1 ½ minutes longer until eggs are completely set.

Substitutions or additions

Mini babybel light ....50 cal.

1 oz. diced canadian bacon ....45 cal.

Egg substitute ....30 cal. per ¼ cup

Diced bell pepper ....10 cal. per ¼ cup chopped

OMELET IN A BAG

This is a quick easy way to make an omelet at home or anywhere... origin unknown...
Girl Scout and campfire favorite!
1 serving @ 150 cal. (basic omelet)

Ingredients

2 large eggs

1 quart size zipper-type resealable plastic bag (freezer weight)

Salt and pepper

Medium-large pot of water heated to a rolling boil

Directions

1. Crack 2 large eggs into plastic bag.

2. Add salt and pepper to taste.

3. Carefully shake and squeeze the eggs in the bag to combine them.

4. Tightly seal the bag, pressing out as much air as possible. The bag should be almost flat.

5. Place the sealed bag into an uncovered pot of rolling boiling water for exactly 13 minutes.

6. Remove bag from water, open the bag, and the omelet will roll out easily.

Note

- You can cook up to 6 omelets in the same large pot of water.
- Add other ingredients in bag with the eggs if desired:

  1 oz. diced canadian bacon . . . . 45 cal.

  Diced bell pepper . . . . 10 cal. per ¼ cup

  Mini Babybel cheese . . . . 50 cal. each

  Laughing Cow Light . . . . 35 cal. per wedge

  2 Tbsp Hormel (real) bacon bits . . . . 50 cal.

CAROL'S FRESH STRAWBERRY PIE
(Adapted from American Heart Association Cookbook; but ingredients changed by me)
8 servings
With Splenda: 139 cal. per serving
With sugar: 187cal. per serving

Ingredients

1 baked pie shell (9 inch) . . . . 100 calories per ⅛ pie

½ cup Splenda . . . . 47.5 cal per ½ cup

  OR sugar . . . . 387 calories per ½ cup

¾ cup of water

2 Tbsp of white corn syrup . . . . 120 cal.

2 Tbsp of corn starch . . . . 61 cal .

1 packet of sugar free or low cal strawberry gelatin powder . . . . 40 cal. per 0.3 ozs.

1 quart* of fresh strawberries washed,

  trimmed and cut in half . . . . 24 cal./cup; approx. 200 cal.

* You may need more depending on their size. It's best to have 2 quarts on hand.

Directions

1. In a saucepan, grind sugar or Splenda with corn starch, using the back of a spoon, until thoroughly mixed.
2. Add water and corn syrup. Bring to a boil and boil for 5 minutes. Stir constantly.
3. Turn off the heat. Add the gelatin powder and stir until thoroughly mixed.
4. Partially cool in fridge.
5. While it cools, arrange the strawberries in the bottom of the baked pie crust. Here is where I eye the pie depth. If it needs to be fuller (depends on the size of strawberries) I add more.
6. Pour the gelatin mixture over the strawberries and chill until set.
7. Serve with cool whip, whipped cream, or whipped cottage cheese (non-fat of course, and remember to count extra calories for the topping).
8. Dust with cinnamon.

JANE'S STAINED GLASS PIE

8 servings @ 168 cal. per serving*

Ingredients

1 small pkg. sugar free cherry jello .... 40 cal.

1 small pkg. sugar free lemon jello .... 40 cal.

1 small pkg. sugar free lime jello .... 40 cal.

1 small pkg. sugar free orange jello .... 40 cal.

1 container (8 ozs.) fat free fat free Cool Whip .... 378 cal.

1 reduced-fat graham cracker pie crust .... 810 cal.

Directions

1. Prepare each package of jello individually in a small, shallow baking dishes, using half the water called for (half cup of boiling water; half cup of cold water).

2. Let the jello set in the refrigerator until hard. Cut each flavor of jello into small squares.

3. Gently mix the multicolored jello squares with the dessert topping.

4. Spoon mixture into the pie crust. Chill and serve.

Note*

- 1348 total cal. with crust
- 10 servings @ 135 cal. per serving
- 538 cal. without crust, served as a dessert in small dish
- 8 servings @ 67 cal. per serving

ROSE'S SALSA
½ cup = 46 calories

Ingredients

2 ½ cups diced peaches

⅓ cup diced red onion

⅓ cup diced red bell pepper

3 Tbsp sliced scallions

3 Tbsp chopped cilantro

3 Tbsp lime juice

Dash salt

Directions

Mix all

CAROL'S FRUIT SMOOTHIE
1 serving @ 195 cal.

Ingredients

6 to 7 ice cubes

1 cup of cold water

½ container of fat free yogurt .... ~40 cal.

½ cup of strawberries, cut up .... 24 cal.

½ cup of blueberries .... 41 cal .

½ banana .... ~45 cal. *depending on the size of the fruit*

½ tsp. almond extract .... negligible

1 Tbsp of Paleo fiber*, vegetable and fruit formula ... Designs for Health, 45 cal.

Directions

Blend until smooth.

Purchased @ New Morning in Woodbury, CT

CARMELA'S ROASTED VEGETABLE DIP
Makes about 16 servings; 4 cups.
Serving size = ¼ cup

Ingredients

2 medium eggplants, peeled and cut into cubes (approx 8 cups) .... 160 cal.

2 medium bell peppers (1 green and 1 red), seeded and cut into 1" pieces .... 60 cal.

1 medium red onion, peeled and cut into 1" pieces .... 50 cal.

2 garlic cloves, minced .... 8 cal.

3 Tbsp olive oil* .... 360 cal.

2 Tbsp tomato paste .... 30 cal.

Salt and pepper to taste .... negligible

Optional: dash cayenne pepper to taste .... negligible

Total approximately 668 cal. or 42 cal. per serving.

Directions

1. Toss the eggplant, bell peppers, onion and garlic in a large bowl with the olive oil. Spread the vegetables in a single layer on a baking sheet. Do not crowd – may need 2 baking sheets. (* NOTE: You can use olive oil cooking spray on baking sheets and vegetables instead of the oil.)

2. Roast at 400 degrees for approx 40 minutes, until the vegetables are lightly browned and soft. Stir at least once during cooking. Remove from oven and allow to cool to room temperature.

3. Place the cooled vegetables in a food processor. Add the tomato paste, and pulse 3 or 4 times to blend but not puree. Leave it slightly chunky. Add salt and black pepper as needed for taste. Add dash of cayenne for heat (optional).

4. Serve with raw vegetables, toasted bread or crackers (count extra calories).

CHAPTER EIGHT

THE BANKING METHOD

REGISTER

Date	Description	Calorie Debit (−)	Calorie Credit (+)	Balance 10,000
10/15	2 eggs			10,000
		140		140
10/15	1 slice of cheese			9,860
		70		70
10/15	2 slices of bread			9,790
		120		120
10/15	1 cup of skim milk			9,670
		90		90
10/15	1 pear			9,600
		90		90
10/15	Treadmill − 40 minutes			9,510
			300	9,810

2,080 calories is the number of calories someone weighing 160 pounds must consume daily in order to maintain that 160 pounds. In order to determine the number of calories you need to maintain your current weight, multiply your weight (up to 200 pounds) by 13. 2,600 calories per day is the cut off point. (200 lbs X 13 = 2,600) You should not be consuming more than 2,600 calories per day for any chance of losing even an ounce.

Once you have established the number of calories you need daily to sustain your weight (and for instructional purposes I will use 2,080 calories per day to maintain a weight of 160 pounds) multiply that number by seven to determine the number of calories per week.

Weight 160 X 13 = 2,080 calories per day
2,080 calories per day X 7 days per week = 14,560 calories per week

Using your banking register, under balance enter your weekly calories (14,560). This is your weekly deposit of calories. Begin entering the number of calories you consume each day, whether it's a meal or snack — whatever you eat. Be diligent. Journal and keep track of those calories. Bank them. Save them. If you "save" 3,500 calories per week you will lose one pound. If you "save" 1,750 calories per week you will lose half a pound. As you enter and "bank" your calories, subtract from the original total you began with. (See the register example above). Make sure you enter exactly what it is you've eaten and the caloric intake. For arguments sake, let's say you consumed 300 calories for breakfast, 275 calories for lunch, 345 calories for dinner, and 365 calories worth of snacks throughout the day you would have banked or saved 1,285 calories that day. Using my weight of 160 pounds and 2,080 calories per week to maintain that weight, if I banked 1,285 calories for a week, a total of 8,995 calories, I would lose approximately 1.5 pounds. 14,560 - 8,995 = 5,565 calories I saved. Remember, if you save 3,500 calories per week, you've lost one pound.

Now let's suppose for a moment I have an occasion to attend the following week, like a wedding that might tempt me to eat something I normally wouldn't consider eating. Well, now I can because I've saved those calories and can use a portion of them for that "special" occasion.

The banking method provides "investments" in health. The "interest" you incur will be the best you ever earned. I saved over $1,200.00 a year in medications I no longer have to take thanks to losing 93 pounds.

If you "overdraft" you make up for it the next day. This is called "banking" your calories. I like to save as many calories as I can healthily during the week so I can enjoy my weekends. NEVER go under 1,200 calories a day.

"Advanced payments" are the bet. I like to save for the weekend before it comes, not after — then it's a penalty.

CHAPTER NINE

DEAR DIARY

*Dear Diary: Friday, Oct. 5, '62. I saw Johnnie in the hall today and he smiled at me!
I was so stupid. I blushed and giggled and ran away to my next class with my girlfriends!*

Oh come on, who didn't have a *Johnnie* in their life? You know, that cute boy with
the letterman sweater, those broad shoulders, "boss" blue eyes, killer smile? Oh those
happy days!

Well, now we're grownups, adults, many of us parents and grandparents and we
don't keep a diary anymore. If we did we'd be able to figure out what happens in our lives
and why we aren't losing weight. After all, that is the point. So if we start to start to write
down whatever we eat, whenever we eat it, we can begin to understand more about ourselves and our eating habits. Even if we begin to journal just a few days a week. Simply
write down what you eat and when you eat it and you'll soon be able to be aware of what's
in front of you and what you are consuming on a daily basis. It's really a stunner - an eye
opener. Sometimes when you do write down your food intake on one specific day, the
next day you're a little bit more careful about what you eat even if you're not writing it
down. It's still a big help and a starting point.

Aside from recording your daily food intake, there are other things you can journal
as well. How about recording your exercise routines each day? I thoroughly enjoy recording my daily exercise routines; it provides me a barometer with which to measure success.
If I walk two miles, I write it down. If I lift weights, I write it down. It gives me a sense
of accomplishment and pride. Journaling my exercise solicits motivation. On days that

I exercise, I did better all around with food intake, as I become more cautious about what I eat. I certainly feel better mentally.

Perhaps a quick entry on what you were feeling that day or what was going on in your life. Was work stressful? Did you accomplish anything positive? Maybe you fell off the wagon. What were your thoughts about that? What time of day were you actually hungry or the hungriest? Many days we aren't that hungry, so why wouldn't we plan out our day by knowing the time of day we are the hungriest? For me, as I kept my diary, I realized that I am a night eater, something I don't think I can change, so I've edited my lifestyle to fit my night eating. I don't eat a lot of breakfast, but I do have a good, hearty, healthy breakfast, usually Fiber One and milk for a total of 150 calories. Same with lunch: a small salad, hard boiled egg and fruit. As a result, I save all my calories for the end of the day, for after five o'clock because that's when I'm going to want my light buttered popcorn, my grapes, my very low in calories strawberry shortcake consisting of sugar free angel food cake, sugar free frozen strawberries, and cool whip. So I've edited my lifestyle but would never have come to this realization had I not kept the diary. I never would have seen where the problem areas existed.

Some people wake up starving, and they should have a hearty, healthy breakfast like a veggie omelet that will keep them going all day long. By making your breakfast your dinner (in terms of calories and when you intake those calories), you've swapped around your day; you've edited your day and your eating habits, and you begin to realize what works best for you. It doesn't matter which meal you edit, but until you start recording it, start using your diary, you won't know what your body needs until you begin.

Another aspect to chronicling your food intake is understanding what foods you like and dislike, need and don't need. When I find a food I like, I just eat it to death! If you keep a diary and record the food that is your favorite, after awhile you just can't stand it. For example, I discovered these very delicious whole wheat pitas consisting of 110 calories each. I started to make refried bean tacos with salsa using the pitas as taco shells. I got so much food for so few calories that I ate them incessantly for days. Eventually, I couldn't stand the sight or smell of another taco and they were eliminated from my menu. Months went by and I was looking for something new and different. I wondered what I had been eating for the past few months that satisfied me so I went to my diary and re-discovered the tacos. Gosh, they were delicious once again. I also started to realize that variety was the spice of life, so I started keeping an area in the back of my journals for favorite foods. I never would have remembered the tacos had I not kept track of what I had been eating. I can't remember half the food I've made, but now I'm going through all my old diaries and finding food I made months, even years ago. It's history. It's all there for me like my own personal recipe book.

Let's say you have a bad week, maybe a couple of bad weeks. It would be great if you could go back and see what you were doing, what you were eating, how you were feeling, how you were exercising during those weeks that were successful. A diary is an excellent tool to help you know yourself and how you can lose weight. You have to design your own healthy lifestyle. You have to design it to fit your needs. Even after losing 93 pounds, I still go back and look at all of my diaries. I will never throw them away, as they are a wealth of information.

PLATEAUS

I had two major plateaus. The first one was at 60 pounds lost. I was on this particular plateau for six months. At the time I could not get past the 60 pound mark. It wasn't until a year later when I was reading the diaries that I realized I thought I looked pretty good. I was off almost all my medicine. I was comfortable. So why lose more weight and get to my goal if I'm happy with the current weight. It became very clear that I was satisfied. I knew that I had to hold the 60 pounds so eventually I moved forward mainly because I started doing a few more baby steps. I could see the same thing happening when I got to my second plateau but thanks to my diary I realized I just had to wait it out till I could move forward. The second plateau was easier to scale thanks to my diary entries. I thought I had attained my goal. I thought I was content, happy and ready for maintenance. I was kidding myself. Yes, I was exercising but using exercise as an excuse to eat more. Would those 60 pounds stay off at this rate? No. My diary was proof that if I was sincere about any further weight loss, I would have to move forward, albeit slowly or regain all that weight I had worked so hard to lose.

Now, I have to laugh at myself. The seriousness and non compromising way I thought I lost weight was really the hard way. Considering the length of time it took me to lose the weight makes me doubt how serious and non compromising I truly was. And therein lies the laugh.

I was lucky. I was such a cheater; losing so little weight each week prepared me for maintenance. Here's the secret, albeit a tad contradictory: cheat! But always be aware of the consequences in your weight loss efforts. Sometimes it is worth it and sometimes it is not. Sometimes it is just necessary.

I couldn't, for the life of me, give up foods I love. I had to make them fit into my healthy new life style. I sort of had to pay for the indulgence. Sometimes I over drafted my account. And yes, there were over draft fees! The two biggest fees I ended up paying were zero weight loss or worse, weight gain. I did learn how to make some of my favorite foods lower in calories and that certainly helped but remember, you can't replace an Espresso Martini!

Re-reading my journals during my weight loss time, I realized that I didn't enjoy the journey. I didn't give myself credit for any of it. If a friend went to the gym, sometimes twice a day, and lost weight steadily I would idolize that friend. But giving credit to myself for even the smallest accomplishment? Not so much.

Realizing my own potential was a daunting task filled with either self doubt or over the top confidence. The journey to self awareness is an ongoing process. Personally, I'm still taking that journey. It's my hope the journey you travel will be as rewarding, as successful, keeping in mind the many potholes, detours and side streets we all have to traverse in order to reach our destination.

Little by little does the trick
~Aesop

Date	Description	Calorie Debit (−)	Calorie Credit (+)	Balance

Activity

_____

_____

Notes

_____

_____

Hold your stomach in at RED Lights-It's makes you look 10 lbs thinner!

Date	Description	Calorie Debit (−)	Calorie Credit (+)	Balance

Activity

_____

_____

_____

Notes

_____

_____

_____

Practice portion control TODAY.

Date	Description	Calorie Debit (−)	Calorie Credit (+)	Balance

Activity

_____

_____

Notes

_____

_____

Just because you have never done something
does not mean you don't have the ability to do it.

Date	Description	Calorie Debit (–)	Calorie Credit (+)	Balance

Activity
_____
_____
_____

Notes
_____
_____
_____

If you focus on results, you will never see change but
if you focus on change, you will see results. ~Connie Wilson

Date	Description	Calorie Debit (−)	Calorie Credit (+)	Balance

Activity

Notes

The best thing about the future is it only comes one day at a time.
~Abraham Lincoln

Date	Description	Calorie Debit (–)	Calorie Credit (+)	Balance

Activity

_____

_____

_____

Notes

_____

_____

_____

DEAR DIARY

Take care of yourself today. Put yourself first.

Date	Description	Calorie Debit (−)	Calorie Credit (+)	Balance

Activity

Notes

Dance like nobody is watching....Eat like everybody is!!!!
~Skinny Week

Date	Description	Calorie Debit (−)	Calorie Credit (+)	Balance

Activity

Notes

Put all your excuses aside and remember this. You are capable.
~Zig Ziglar

Date	Description	Calorie Debit (−)	Calorie Credit (+)	Balance

Activity

Notes

Treat yourself like company.

Date	Description	Calorie Debit (−)	Calorie Credit (+)	Balance

Activity

_____

_____

Notes

_____

_____

You can't lose weight one way and keep it off another.

Date	Description	Calorie Debit (−)	Calorie Credit (+)	Balance

Activity

Notes

The achievement of one goal should be the starting point of another
~Alexander Graham Bell

Date	Description	Calorie Debit (−)	Calorie Credit (+)	Balance

Activity

_____

_____

_____

Notes

_____

_____

_____

To eat is a neccessity, but to eat intelligently is an art
~La rochefoucauld

Date	Description	Calorie Debit (−)	Calorie Credit (+)	Balance

Activity

Notes

You must begin to think of yourself as becoming the person you want to be
~David Viscott

Date	Description	Calorie Debit (−)	Calorie Credit (+)	Balance

Activity

_____

_____

Notes

_____

_____

Our greatest glory is not in never failing, but in rising every time we fall
~Confucious

Date	Description	Calorie Debit (−)	Calorie Credit (+)	Balance

Activity

Notes

Clear your mind of CAN'T
~Dr. Samuel Johnson

Date	Description	Calorie Debit (−)	Calorie Credit (+)	Balance

Activity
_____
_____
_____

Notes
_____
_____
_____

You've got to say, I think that if I keep working at this and want it badly enough, I can have it. It's called perserverance   ~Lee Iacocca

Date	Description	Calorie Debit (−)	Calorie Credit (+)	Balance

Activity

_____

_____

_____

Notes

_____

_____

_____

The difference between try and triumph is just a little umph
~Marvin Phillips

Date	Description	Calorie Debit (−)	Calorie Credit (+)	Balance

Activity

Notes

Success is not the result of spontaneous combustion, You must set yourself on fire
~Reggie leach

Date	Description	Calorie Debit (−)	Calorie Credit (+)	Balance

Activity

_____

_____

Notes

_____

_____

You only have to write down your food intake
on the days you want to lose weight.

Date	Description	Calorie Debit (−)	Calorie Credit (+)	Balance

Activity
_____
_____
_____

Notes
_____
_____
_____

Take care of your body, it is the only place you have to live
~Jim Rohn

Date	Description	Calorie Debit (−)	Calorie Credit (+)	Balance

Activity

Notes

Don't feed the mood with food.

Date	Description	Calorie Debit (−)	Calorie Credit (+)	Balance

Activity

Notes

We never repent of having eaten too little
~Thomas Jefferson

Date	Description	Calorie Debit (–)	Calorie Credit (+)	Balance

Activity

_____

_____

_____

Notes

_____

_____

_____

Treat yourself to something special today.

Date	Description	Calorie Debit (−)	Calorie Credit (+)	Balance

Activity

_____

_____

_____

Notes

_____

_____

_____

Are you holding your stomach in at red lights?

Date	Description	Calorie Debit (−)	Calorie Credit (+)	Balance

Activity

Notes

What can I do to make myself a priorty today?

Date	Description	Calorie Debit (–)	Calorie Credit (+)	Balance

Activity

_____

_____

_____

Notes

_____

_____

_____

Would you rather wear anything you want or eat anything you want?

Date	Description	Calorie Debit (−)	Calorie Credit (+)	Balance

Activity

_____

_____

Notes

_____

_____

Don't diet, EDIT!

Date	Description	Calorie Debit (−)	Calorie Credit (+)	Balance

Activity

Notes

Rather than aiming to be perfect, aim to be just a little better today.

Date	Description	Calorie Debit (−)	Calorie Credit (+)	Balance

Activity

Notes

Don't exchange what you want most for what you want at the moment.

Date	Description	Calorie Debit (−)	Calorie Credit (+)	Balance

Activity

_____

_____

Notes

_____

_____

Don't let your meals say "I am on a diet".

Date	Description	Calorie Debit (−)	Calorie Credit (+)	Balance

Activity

Notes

Don't put food in your mouth when you have food in your mouth.

Date	Description	Calorie Debit (−)	Calorie Credit (+)	Balance

Activity

Notes

Stand up straight. You will look 10 pounds thinner.

Date	Description	Calorie Debit (−)	Calorie Credit (+)	Balance

Activity

Notes

Nothing tastes as good as being thin feels.

Date	Description	Calorie Debit (−)	Calorie Credit (+)	Balance

Activity

Notes

What is one small step you are willing to take today to move forward?

Date	Description	Calorie Debit (−)	Calorie Credit (+)	Balance

Activity

Notes

Observe your comfort zone.

Date	Description	Calorie Debit (−)	Calorie Credit (+)	Balance

Activity

_____

_____

Notes

_____

_____

DEAR DIARY

Stay ahead of hunger.

Date	Description	Calorie Debit (-)	Calorie Credit (+)	Balance

Activity

Notes

Seven days without activity makes one 'weak'.

Date	Description	Calorie Debit (–)	Calorie Credit (+)	Balance

Activity

_____

_____

Notes

_____

_____

Notice *all* progress.

Date	Description	Calorie Debit (−)	Calorie Credit (+)	Balance

Activity

Notes

Look back and learn.

Date	Description	Calorie Debit (−)	Calorie Credit (+)	Balance

Activity

_____

_____

Notes

_____

_____

Variety is the spice of life, try something new today.

Date	Description	Calorie Debit (−)	Calorie Credit (+)	Balance

Activity

Notes

Don't sabotage yourself.

Date	Description	Calorie Debit (−)	Calorie Credit (+)	Balance

Activity

_____

_____

Notes

_____

_____

When faced with a challenge, lost for a way, not a way out
~David Weatherford

Date	Description	Calorie Debit (−)	Calorie Credit (+)	Balance

Activity

Notes

Let our advance worrying become our advance thinking and planning
~Winston Churchhill

Date	Description	Calorie Debit (−)	Calorie Credit (+)	Balance

Activity

Notes

Persistance: Everyone starts from scratch but not everyone keeps scratching.

Date	Description	Calorie Debit (–)	Calorie Credit (+)	Balance

Activity

_____

_____

_____

Notes

_____

_____

_____

The harder you work, the harder it is to surrender
~Vince Lomardi

Date	Description	Calorie Debit (−)	Calorie Credit (+)	Balance

Activity
_____
_____
_____

Notes
_____
_____
_____

Don't go for all or nothing, go for a little something something
~Cherie Blessum

Date	Description	Calorie Debit (−)	Calorie Credit (+)	Balance

Activity

_____

_____

_____

Notes

_____

_____

_____

Your past does not equal, nor does it dictate, your future.

Date	Description	Calorie Debit (−)	Calorie Credit (+)	Balance

Activity

_____

_____

Notes

_____

_____

One definition of insanity is:
Doing the same thing again and again and expecting a different result.

Date	Description	Calorie Debit (−)	Calorie Credit (+)	Balance

Activity

Notes

Your past does not equal, nor does it dictate, your future.

Date	Description	Calorie Debit (−)	Calorie Credit (+)	Balance

Activity

_____

_____

Notes

_____

_____

Do you choose to simply know the path, or do you choose to walk it?

Date	Description	Calorie Debit (−)	Calorie Credit (+)	Balance

Activity

_____

_____

Notes

_____

_____

Rather than aiming for being perfect,
just aim to be little bit better today than you were yesterday.

Date	Description	Calorie Debit (−)	Calorie Credit (+)	Balance

Activity

Notes

Discipline is remembering what you want.

Date	Description	Calorie Debit (−)	Calorie Credit (+)	Balance

Activity

Notes

Your body keeps an accurate journal regardless of what you write down...

Date	Description	Calorie Debit (−)	Calorie Credit (+)	Balance

Activity

_____

_____

_____

Notes

_____

_____

_____

Every time you are tempted to react in the same old way, ask if you want to be a prisoner of the past or a pioneer of the future. ~Deepak Chopra

Date	Description	Calorie Debit (−)	Calorie Credit (+)	Balance

Activity

_____

_____

_____

Notes

_____

_____

_____

A year from now, you may wish you had started today
~Robert Schuller

Date	Description	Calorie Debit (−)	Calorie Credit (+)	Balance

Activity
_____
_____
_____

Notes
_____
_____
_____

"Our greatest glory is not in never falling, but in rising every time we fall" ~confucious

Date	Description	Calorie Debit (−)	Calorie Credit (+)	Balance

Activity

Notes

Never, never, never, never give up.
~Winston Churchill

Date	Description	Calorie Debit (−)	Calorie Credit (+)	Balance

Activity

_____

_____

Notes

_____

_____

Rule your mind or it will rule you.
~Horace

Date	Description	Calorie Debit (−)	Calorie Credit (+)	Balance

Activity

Notes

You've got to say, I think that if I keep working at this and want it badly enough I can have it. It's called perseverance. ~Lee Iacocca

Date	Description	Calorie Debit (−)	Calorie Credit (+)	Balance

Activity

_____

_____

Notes

_____

_____

The first and the best victory is to conquer self.
~Plato

Date	Description	Calorie Debit (−)	Calorie Credit (+)	Balance

Activity

Notes

The road to success is dotted with many tempting parking places.
~Unknown

Date	Description	Calorie Debit (–)	Calorie Credit (+)	Balance

Activity

Notes

The time for action is now. It's never too late to do something.
~Carl Sandburg

Date	Description	Calorie Debit (−)	Calorie Credit (+)	Balance

Activity

Notes

"Bigger snacks mean bigger slacks."
~Unknown

Date	Description	Calorie Debit (−)	Calorie Credit (+)	Balance

Activity
_____
_____
_____

Notes
_____
_____
_____

It's not the minutes spent at the table that put on weight, it's the seconds.

Date	Description	Calorie Debit (–)	Calorie Credit (+)	Balance

Activity

Notes

"I've been on a diet for two weeks and all I've lost is two weeks."
~Totie Fields

Date	Description	Calorie Debit (−)	Calorie Credit (+)	Balance

Activity
_____
_____
_____

Notes
_____
_____
_____

"Action is the foundational key to all success."
~Pablo Picasso

Date	Description	Calorie Debit (−)	Calorie Credit (+)	Balance

Activity

_____

_____

Notes

_____

_____

"No matter who you are, no matter what you do, you absolutely, positively do have the power to change." ~Bill Phillips

Date	Description	Calorie Debit (-)	Calorie Credit (+)	Balance

Activity

Notes

"You must begin to think of yourself as becoming the person you want to be." ~David Viscott

Date	Description	Calorie Debit (−)	Calorie Credit (+)	Balance

Activity

Notes

"No matter who you are, no matter what you do, you absolutely, positively do have the power to change." ~Bill Phillips

Date	Description	Calorie Debit (−)	Calorie Credit (+)	Balance

Activity

Notes

"You must begin to think of yourself as becoming the person
you want to be." ~David Viscott

Date	Description	Calorie Debit (−)	Calorie Credit (+)	Balance

Activity

Notes

Little by little does the trick
~Aesop

Date	Description	Calorie Debit (−)	Calorie Credit (+)	Balance

Activity
_____
_____
_____

Notes
_____
_____
_____

Hold your stomach in at RED Lights–It's makes you look 10 lbs thinner!

Date	Description	Calorie Debit (−)	Calorie Credit (+)	Balance

Activity

Notes

Practice portion control TODAY

Date	Description	Calorie Debit (−)	Calorie Credit (+)	Balance

Activity

Notes

Just because you have never done something
does not mean you don't have the ability to do it.

Date	Description	Calorie Debit (−)	Calorie Credit (+)	Balance

Activity

Notes

If you focus on results, you will never see change but
if you focus on change, you will see results. ~Connie Wilson

Date	Description	Calorie Debit (−)	Calorie Credit (+)	Balance

Activity

Notes

The best thing about the future is it only comes once day at a time.
~Abraham Lincoln

Date	Description	Calorie Debit (−)	Calorie Credit (+)	Balance

Activity

_____

_____

Notes

_____

_____

Take care of yourself today. Put yourself first.

Date	Description	Calorie Debit (−)	Calorie Credit (+)	Balance

Activity

Notes

Dance like nobody is watching....Eat like everybody is!!!!
~Skinny Week

Date	Description	Calorie Debit (-)	Calorie Credit (+)	Balance

Activity

_____

_____

Notes

_____

_____

Put all your excuses aside and remember this. You are capable.
~Zig Ziglar

Date	Description	Calorie Debit (-)	Calorie Credit (+)	Balance

Activity
_____
_____
_____

Notes
_____
_____
_____

Treat yourself like company.

Date	Description	Calorie Debit (−)	Calorie Credit (+)	Balance

Activity

Notes

You can't lose weight one way and keep it off another.

Date	Description	Calorie Debit (−)	Calorie Credit (+)	Balance

Activity

_____

_____

Notes

_____

_____

DEAR DIARY

The achievement of one goal should be the starting point of another
~Alexander Graham Bell

Date	Description	Calorie Debit (−)	Calorie Credit (+)	Balance

Activity

Notes

To eat is a neccessity, but to eat intelligently is an art
~La rochefoucauld

Date	Description	Calorie Debit (−)	Calorie Credit (+)	Balance

Activity

Notes

You must begin to think of yourself as to become the person you want to be
~David Viscott

Date	Description	Calorie Debit (−)	Calorie Credit (+)	Balance

Activity
_____
_____
_____

Notes
_____
_____
_____

Our greatest glory is not in never failing, but in rising every time we fall
~Confucious

Date	Description	Calorie Debit (−)	Calorie Credit (+)	Balance

Activity

Notes

Clear your mind of CAN'T
~Dr. Samuel Johnson

Date	Description	Calorie Debit (−)	Calorie Credit (+)	Balance

Activity

Notes

You've got to say, nI think that if I keep working at this and want it badly enough, I can have it. It's called perserverance   ~Lee Iacocca

Date	Description	Calorie Debit (−)	Calorie Credit (+)	Balance

Activity

Notes

The difference between try and triumph is just a little umph
~Marvin Phillips

Date	Description	Calorie Debit (−)	Calorie Credit (+)	Balance

Activity

_____

_____

_____

Notes

_____

_____

_____

Success is not the result of spontaneous combustion, You must set yourself on fire
~Reggie leach

Date	Description	Calorie Debit (-)	Calorie Credit (+)	Balance

Activity

_____

_____

Notes

_____

_____

You only have to write down your food intake
on the days you want to lose weight.

Date	Description	Calorie Debit (−)	Calorie Credit (+)	Balance

Activity

Notes

Take care of your body, it is the only place you have to live
~Jim Rohn

Date	Description	Calorie Debit (−)	Calorie Credit (+)	Balance

Activity

Notes

Don't feed the mood with food.

Date	Description	Calorie Debit (−)	Calorie Credit (+)	Balance

Activity
_____
_____
_____

Notes
_____
_____
_____

We never repent of having eaten too little
~Thomas Jefferson

Date	Description	Calorie Debit (−)	Calorie Credit (+)	Balance

Activity

_____

_____

_____

Notes

_____

_____

_____

Treat yourself to something special today.

Date	Description	Calorie Debit (−)	Calorie Credit (+)	Balance

Activity

Notes

Are you holding your stomach in at red lights?

Date	Description	Calorie Debit (−)	Calorie Credit (+)	Balance

Activity

_____

_____

_____

Notes

_____

_____

_____

What can I do to make myself a priorty today?

Date	Description	Calorie Debit (−)	Calorie Credit (+)	Balance

Activity

_____

_____

_____

Notes

_____

_____

_____

Would you rather wear anything you want or eat anything you want?

Date	Description	Calorie Debit (−)	Calorie Credit (+)	Balance

Activity

Notes

Don't diet, EDIT!

Date	Description	Calorie Debit (-)	Calorie Credit (+)	Balance

Activity

Notes

Rather than aiming to be perfect, aim to be just a little better today.

Date	Description	Calorie Debit (−)	Calorie Credit (+)	Balance

Activity
_____
_____
_____

Notes
_____
_____
_____

Don't exchange what you want most for what you want at the moment.

Date	Description	Calorie Debit (−)	Calorie Credit (+)	Balance

Activity

_____

_____

_____

Notes

_____

_____

_____

Don't let your meals say "I am on a diet".

Date	Description	Calorie Debit (-)	Calorie Credit (+)	Balance

Activity

_____

Notes

_____

Don't put food in your mouth when you have food in your mouth.

Date	Description	Calorie Debit (−)	Calorie Credit (+)	Balance

Activity

_____

_____

Notes

_____

_____

Stand up straight. You will look 10 pounds thinner.

Date	Description	Calorie Debit (−)	Calorie Credit (+)	Balance

Activity

Notes

Nothing tastes as good as being thin feels.

Date	Description	Calorie Debit (-)	Calorie Credit (+)	Balance

Activity

Notes

What is one small step you are willing to take today to move forward?

Date	Description	Calorie Debit (-)	Calorie Credit (+)	Balance

Activity

Notes

www.ingramcontent.com/pod-product-compliance
Lightning Source LLC
Chambersburg PA
CBHW060252290526
45789CB00001B/302